RECOGNITION AND
MANAGEMENT OF
PESTICIDE POISONINGS

Fifth Edition, 1999

J. Routt Reigart, M.D.
Professor of Pediatrics, Medical University of South Carolina

James R. Roberts, M.D., M.P.H.
Assistant Professor of Pediatrics, Medical University of South Carolina

Support for this publication was provided by:
Certification and Worker Protection Branch
Field and External Affairs Division
Office of Pesticide Programs
U.S. Environmental Protection Agency
401 M Street SW (7506C)
Washington, DC 20460

For additional copies or more information:
Tel: 703–305–7666
Fax: 703–308–2962

The manual is available in electronic format on the Internet at:
http://www.epa.gov/pesticides/safety/healthcare

Acknowledgments

We are grateful to the Office of Pesticide Programs, Environmental Protection Agency, for giving us the opportunity to collaborate on this new edition. Our thanks go to Kevin Keaney, Acting Branch Chief, for his support and vision, and for giving this publication priority attention. Particular mention should also be made of the efforts of Jerome M. Blondell, Ph.D., M.P.H., and Ameesha Mehta, M.P.H., whose oversight and constant assistance were invaluable in moving this project forward. Ana Maria Osorio, M.D., M.P.H., contributed Chapter 3, Environmental and Occupational History, to this manual.

Experts in clinical toxicology conducted critical reviews of draft material. We are greatly appreciative of the time and effort of the following reviewers:

Jeffery Lloyd Burgess, M.D., M.P.H.
Assistant Professor
Environmental Occupational Health Unit
University of Arizona Prevention Center

Matthew C. Keifer, M.D., M.P.H.
Assistant Professor
Department of Medicine/Environmental Health
University of Washington

Wayne R. Snodgrass, M.D., Ph.D.
Professor and Head
Clinical Pharmacology-Toxicology
Texas Poison Center

Sheldon L. Wagner, M.D.
Professor of Clinical Toxicology
Oregon State University

Many other individuals contributed their time and skill to this publication. We are very appreciative of the tireless efforts of Patricia Clark, our administrative assistant, who spent endless hours in text review, securing references, communicating with reviewers, and otherwise making the revision process possible and easier than anticipated. Gilah Langner of Stretton Associates, Inc., provided editorial supervision. Will Packard and Sarah Carter of Free Hand Press, Inc. were responsible for the format and layout of the manual.

Cover photographs by Steve Delaney, EPA.

CONTENTS

List of Tables

Dosage Tables

Tables

Section I

GENERAL INFORMATION

CHAPTER 1

Introduction

This fifth edition of *Recognition and Management of Pesticide Poisonings* is an update and expansion of the 1989 fourth edition. The Office of Pesticide Programs of the United States Environmental Protection Agency has sponsored the series since 1973. The purpose of the manual is to provide health professionals with recently available information on the health hazards of pesticides currently in use, and current consensus recommendations for management of poisonings and injuries caused by them.

Pesticide poisoning is a commonly under-diagnosed illness in America today. Despite recommendations by the Institute of Medicine and others urging the integration of environmental medicine into medical education, health care providers generally receive a very limited amount of training in occupational and environmental health, and in pesticide-related illnesses, in particular.[1] The updating of this manual is part of a larger initiative of the U.S. Environmental Protection Agency, in conjunction with numerous federal agencies, associations of health professionals, and related organizations to help health care providers become better aware, educated, and trained in the area of pesticide-related health concerns. This larger initiative, entitled Pesticides and National Strategies for Health Care Providers, was launched in April 1998.

As with previous updates, this new edition incorporates new pesticide products that are not necessarily widely known among health professionals. The accumulated "use experience" of formulators, applicators, and field workers provides an expanding basis for judging safety and identifying the environmental and workplace hazards of old and new pesticides. Major episodes of adverse health effects reported in medical and scientific periodicals have been taken into account. This literature also contributes importantly to improved understanding of toxic mechanisms. Clinical toxicology is a dynamic field of medicine; new treatment methods are developed regularly, and the effectiveness of old as well as new modalities is subject to constant critical review.

There is general agreement that *prevention* of pesticide poisoning remains a much surer path to safety and health than reliance on treatment. In addition to the inherent toxicity of pesticides, none of the medical procedures or drugs used in treating poisonings is risk-free. In fact, many antidotes are toxic in their own right, and such apparently simple procedures as gastric intubation incur substantial risk. The clinical toxicologist must often weigh the hazards of various courses of action—sometimes including no treatment at all—against the risks of various interventions, such as gastric emptying, catharsis, administration of intravenous fluids, or administration of an antidote, if available. Clinical management decisions have to be made promptly and, as often as not, on the basis of limited scientific and medical information. The complex circumstances of human poisonings rarely allow precise comparisons of alternative management. In no sense, then, are the treatment recommendations in this book infallible guides to successful outcomes. They are no more than consensus judgments of the best available clinical management options.

This manual deals almost entirely with short-term (acute) harmful effects of pesticides. Although obviously important, the subject of chronic effects is too complex to deal with exhaustively in a manual designed as guidance for emergency management. Nonetheless, appropriate treatment of serious exposures to pesticides represents an important step in avoiding chronic as well as acute disease.

The pesticides and commercial products mentioned in this manual do not represent the universe of pesticide products in existence. They were selected based on frequency of use and exposure, severity of toxicity, and prior experience with acute poisonings. Products are discussed in this manual that have been discontinued or whose U.S. pesticide registration has been revoked but are judged to still be of risk due to use elsewhere or where there is a probability of residual stocks. Agents long out of use in the U.S. and elsewhere were not included in the manual.

The amount of pesticide absorbed is a critical factor in making treatment decisions, and estimation of dosage in many circumstances of pesticide exposure remains difficult. The terms "small amount" and "large amount" used in this book are obviously ambiguous, but the quality of exposure information obtained rarely justifies more specific terminology.

Sometimes the circumstances of exposure are a rough guide to the amount absorbed. Exposure to spray drift properly diluted for field application is not likely to convey a large dose unless exposure has been prolonged. Spills of concentrated technical material onto the skin or clothing may well represent a large dose of pesticide unless the contamination is promptly removed. Brief dermal exposure to foliage residues of cholinesterase-inhibiting pesticides is not likely to lead to poisoning, but prolonged exposures may well do so. Suicidal ingestions almost always involve "large amounts," requiring the most aggressive management. Except in children, accidental pesticide ingestions are likely to be spat out or vomited. Ingestions of pesticides by children are the most difficult to evaluate. The therapist usually must base clinical management decisions on "worst case" assumptions of dosage. Childhood poisonings are still further complicated by the greater vulnerability of the very young, not only to pesticides themselves, but also to drugs and treatment procedures. The nature of neurological development in children entails an additional level of risk that is not present in adults. Some adult groups such as farmwrokers with poor nutrition and high exposure may also be at increased risk.

Key Principles

General methods of managing pesticide poisonings are presented in Chapter 2 and reflect a broad base of clinical experience. The following key points deserve emphasis. The need to protect the airway from aspiration of vomitus cannot be overstated. Death has occasionally resulted from this complication, even following ingestions of substances having relatively low toxic potential. In poisonings by agents that depress central nervous system function or cause convulsions, early placement of a cuffed endotracheal tube (even when this requires light general anesthesia) may be life saving. Maintenance of adequate pulmonary gas exchange is another essential element of poisoning management that deserves constant reemphasis.

Gastric intubation, with aspiration and lavage, remains a useful method for removing poisons from the stomach shortly after they have been swallowed, but the time after ingestion during which lavage is likely to be beneficial is shorter than many clinical toxicologists have thought. Rarely are significant amounts of swallowed toxicants recovered more than 1-2 hours after ingestion, and, in many instances, the bulk of swallowed material passes into the duodenum and beyond in 15-30 minutes. In addition, the majority of controlled studies evaluating the effectiveness of gastric emptying procedures are done for ingestions of solid material (pills) rather than liquids.

Full advantage should be taken of new highly adsorbent charcoals that are effective in binding some pesticides in the gut. Unfortunately, charcoal does not adsorb all pesticides, and its efficiency against many of them is not known. In poisonings caused by large intakes of pesticide, hemodialysis and hemoperfusion over adsorbents continue to be tested as methods for reducing body burdens. Against some toxicants, these procedures appear valuable. Overall effectiveness appears to depend not only on efficiency of clearance from the blood, but also on the mobility of toxicant already distributed to tissues before the extracorporeal blood-purification procedure is started. The volume of distribution and avidity of tissue binding are important considerations in making such decisions. The critical determinant of success in using these systems may well be the speed with which they can be put into operation before tissue-damaging stores of toxicant have accumulated.

There remains a need for systematic reporting of pesticide poisonings to a central agency so that accurate statistics describing the frequency and circumstances of poisoning can be compiled, and efforts to limit these occurrences can be properly directed. In some countries there has been an increase in the use of pesticides as instruments of suicide and even homicide. Producers are now devoting considerable effort to modifying formulation and packaging to deter these misuses. This work is important because suicidal ingestions are often the most difficult pesticide poisonings to treat successfully.

Common Pesticide Poisonings

The pesticides most often implicated in poisonings, injuries, and illnesses, according to 1996 data from the American Association of Poison Control Center's Toxic Exposure Surveillance System, are listed below.

The list is based on symptomatic cases classified as minor, moderate, major, or fatal outcome for unintentional cases involving a single product. Numbers of cases are reported for both children under six years of age and for adults and older children. Suicide/homicide (intentional) cases have been excluded. Cases listed as organophosphates (and the other categories as well) may also include other insecticides such as carbamates and organochlorines in a single product.

PESTICIDES MOST OFTEN IMPLICATED IN SYMPTOMATIC ILLNESSES, 1996

Rank	Pesticide or Pesticide Class	Child < 6 years	Adults 6-19 yrs.	Total*
1	Organophosphates	700	3274	4002
2	Pyrethrins and pyrethroids**	1100	2850	3950
3	Pine oil disinfectants	1336	903	2246
4	Hypochlorite disinfectants	808	1291	2109
5	Insect repellents	1081	997	2086
6	Phenol disinfectants	630	405	1040
7	Carbamate insecticides	202	817	1030
8	Organochlorine insecticides	229	454	685
9	Phenoxy herbicides	63	387	453
10	Anticoagulant rodenticides	176	33	209
	All Other Pesticides	954	3604	4623
	Total all pesticides/disinfectants	7279	15,015	22,433

* Totals include a small number of cases with unknown age.
** Rough estimate: includes some veterinary products not classified by chemical type.

Source: American Association of Poison Control Centers, Toxic Exposure Surveillance System, 1996 data.

Approximately 90% of symptomatic cases involve only minor symptoms of the type that could typically be treated at home with dilution or just observation. However, seven of the top ten categories listed in the table above (organophosphates, pyrethrins/pyrethroids, hypochlorite disinfectants, carbamates, organochlorines, phenoxy herbicides, and anticoagulant rodenticides) are much more likely to require medical attention.

This list cannot be considered representative of all symptomatic poisonings because it only shows cases reported to Poison Control Centers. However, it does give a sense of the relative frequency and risk of poisoning from various agents or classes of agents. The relative frequency of cases generally reflects how widely a product is used in the environment. For example, a number of disinfectants occur in the top ten partly because they are far more commonly found in the home and work environment than other pesticides (see also the table of occupational cases below). Denominator information on the population at risk (numbers exposed) would be needed to better understand the relative risk of different pesticides. However, the main purpose of these tables is to give physicians a sense of what types of cases they are most likely to see in their practice.

Although suicide cases make up roughly 3% of pesticide-related calls to Poison Control Centers, they may account for nearly 10% of the cases seen in a health care facility. The leading types of products involved in suicidal cases include anticoagulant rodenticides (20% of total suicide attempts), pine oil disinfectants (14%), organophosphates (11%), pyrethrins/pyrethroids (6%), unknown rodenticides (5%), carbamate insecticides (4%), and phenol disinfectants (3%).

CALIFORNIA OCCUPATIONAL ILLNESSES LIKELY DUE TO PESTICIDES, 1991-1995

Rank	Pesticide	Systemic	Topical*	Total
1	Sodium hypochlorite	167	858	1025
2	Quaternary ammonia	9	348	357
3	Chlorine	112	124	236
4	Glutaraldehyde	38	118	156
5	Chlorpyrifos	113	39	152
6	Sulfur	48	69	117
7	Glyphosate	9	94	103
8	Propargite	3	96	99
9	Metam sodium**	64	33	97
10	Cyanuric acid	14	76	90
	All Other	1149	1089	2238
	Total all pesticides/disinfectants	1726	2944	4670

* Topical includes skin, eye, and respiratory effects.
** Train derailment led to a cluster of cases due to metam sodium in 1991.

Source: Louise Mehler, M.S., California Pesticide Illness Surveillance Program, California Environmental Protection Agency.

Poison Control Centers are best at capturing pesticide exposures which occur in residential environments. However, occupational exposures are not as well covered. California's Pesticide Illness Surveillance Program is generally regarded as the best in the country. The table above presents the number of occupationally-related cases in California reported from 1991 through 1995 where a pesticide was considered a probable or definite cause of the resulting illness. Pesticide combinations, where the primary pesticide responsible for the illness could not be identified, are not included in this table. Among persons who encounter pesticides in the course of their occupational activities, dermal and eye injuries, rather than systemic poisonings, are more common. Systemic poisonings, however, are likely to be more severe.

Format of this Manual

An effort has been made to format this book for quick reference by thorough indexing and minimal references to other pages or chapters. However, many different agents commonly require similar procedures in treating poisonings and it is not practical to repeat these protocols in every chapter. General principles for management of pesticide poisoning, including skin and eye decontamination, gastrointestinal decontamination, and control of convulsions are considered in Chapter 2, General Principles. These principles are referenced throughout.

Changes in this reformatted edition include: tabular listings of Commercial Products in each chapter, the addition of a new chapter on Disinfectants (Chapter 19), and the addition of a chapter on Environmental and Occupational History (Chapter 3), which places pesticide poisonings in the context of other environmental and occupational exposures, provides questionnaires designed to elicit exposure information, discusses resources available to the practitioner, and provides a list of governmental and non-government contacts and Web sites for more information. In addition, each chapter is referenced to key references in readily accessible current literature. Most references were selected as primary references in peer review journals, although some review papers are also included.

The contents of this book have been derived from many sources: published texts, current medical, toxicological, and pesticide product literature, and direct communications with experts in clinical toxicology and pesticide toxicology and environmental and occupational health specialists. A list of the major text sources follows this introduction.

Reference

1. Institute of Medicine. Role of the Primary Care Physician in Occupational and Environmental Medicine, Washington, DC: Institute of Medicine, 1988.

Texts and Handbooks on Pesticides, Pesticide Toxicology, and Clinical Toxicology

Agricultural Chemicals Books I, II, III, IV
W. T. Thomson
Thomson Publications, Fresno, CA, 1994-95

Agrochemicals Desk Reference: Environmental Data
John H. Montgomery
Lewis Publishers, Boca Raton, FL, 1995

The Agrochemicals Handbook, 3rd Edition
The Royal Society of Chemistry, Cambridge, England, 1994

**Biological Monitoring Methods for Industrial Chemicals,
2nd Edition**
Randall C. Baselt
Biomedical Publications, Davis, CA, 1988

Casarett and Doull's Toxicology, 5th Edition
John Doull, Curtis D. Klaassen, and Mary O. Amdur
Macmillan Publishing Company, New York, NY, 1996

Chemicals Identified in Human Biological Media: A Data Base
Compiled by M. Virginia Cone, Margaret F. Baldauf, Fay M. Martin, and John
    T. Ensminger
Oak Ridge National Laboratory, 1980

Clinical Toxicology of Agricultural Chemicals
Sheldon L. Wagner, M.D.
Oregon State University Press, Corvallis, OR, 1981

Clinical Toxicology of Commercial Products, 5th Edition
Robert E. Gosselin, Roger P. Smith and Harold C. Hodge, with assistance of
    Jeannette E. Braddock
Williams and Wilkins, Baltimore, MD, 1984

Farm Chemicals Handbook
Charlotte Sine, Editorial Director
Meister Publishing Company, Willoughby, Ohio, 1998

Handbook of Pesticide Toxicology
Wayland J. Hayes, Jr. and Edward R. Laws, Jr., Editors
Academic Press, San Diego, CA 1991

**Handbook of Poisoning: Prevention, Diagnosis and Treatment,
12th Edition**
Robert H. Dreisbach and William O. Robertson
Appleton and Lange, East Norwalk, CT, 1987

Herbicide Handbook, 7th Edition
Weed Science Society of America, 1994

Medical Toxicology: Diagnosis and Treatment of Human Poisoning
Matthew J. Ellenhorn and Donald G. Barceloux
Elsevier, New York, NY, 1988

The Merck Index, 11th Edition
Martha Windholz and Susan Budavari, Editors
Merck and Company, Inc., Rahway, NJ, 1989

Patty's Industrial Hygiene and Toxicology, 4th Revised Edition
George D. Clayton and Florence E. Clayton
Wiley Interscience, New York, NY, 1991–95

Pesticide Manual, 11th Edition
CDS Tomlin
The British Crop Protection Council, Farnham, Surrey, United Kingdom, 1997

Pesticide Profiles: Toxicity, Environmental Impact, and Fate
Michael A. Kamrin (Editor)
Lewis Publishers, Boca Raton, FL, 1997

The Pharmacological Basis of Therapeutics, 8th Edition
Louis S. Goodman and Alfred Gilman
Pergamon Press, New York, NY, 1990

POISINDEX® System
Barry H. Rumack, N.K. Sayre, and C.R. Gelman, Editors
Micromedex, Englewood, CO, 1974–98

Poisoning: A Guide to Clinical Diagnosis and Treatment, 2nd Edition
W. F. Von Oettingen
W. B. Saunders Company, Philadelphia, PA, 1958

CHAPTER 2

General Principles in the Management of Acute Pesticide Poisonings

This chapter describes basic management techniques applicable to most acute pesticide poisonings. Where special considerations and treatments are required for a particular pesticide, they are addressed separately in the appropriate chapter.

Skin Decontamination

Decontamination must proceed concurrently with whatever resuscitative and antidotal measures are necessary to preserve life. Shower patient with soap and water, and shampoo hair to remove chemicals from skin and hair. If there are any indications of weakness, ataxia, or other neurologic impairment, clothing should be removed and a complete bath and shampoo given while the victim is recumbent. The possibility of pesticide sequestered under fingernails or in skin folds should not be overlooked.

Flush contaminating chemicals from eyes with copious amounts of clean water for 10-15 minutes. If eye irritation is present after decontamination, ophthalmologic consultation is appropriate.

Persons attending the victim should avoid direct contact with heavily contaminated clothing and vomitus. Contaminated clothing should be promptly removed, bagged, and laundered before returning. Shoes and other leather items cannot usually be decontaminated and should be discarded. Note that pesticides can contaminate the inside surfaces of gloves, boots, and headgear. Decontamination should especially be considered for emergency personnel such as ambulance drivers at the site of a spill or contamination. Wear rubber gloves while washing pesticide from skin and hair of patient. Latex and other surgical or precautionary gloves usually will not always adequately protect from pesticide contamination, so only rubber gloves are appropriate for this purpose.

Airway Protection

Ensure that a clear airway exists. Suction any oral secretions using a large bore suction device if necessary. Intubate the trachea if the patient has respiratory depression or if the patient appears obtunded or otherwise neurologically impaired. Administer oxygen as necessary to maintain adequate tissue oxygenation. In severe poisonings, it may be necessary to mechanically support pulmonary ventilation for several days.

Note on Specific Pesticides: There are several special considerations with regard to certain pesticides. In **organophosphate** and **carbamate** poisoning, adequate tissue oxygenation is essential prior to administering atropine. As important, in **paraquat** and **diquat** poisoning, oxygen is **contraindicated** early in the poisoning because of progressive oxygen toxicity to the lung tissue. See specific chapters for more details.

Gastrointestinal Decontamination

A joint position statement has recently been released by the American Academy of Clinical Toxicology and the European Association of Poisons Centres and Clinical Toxicologists on various methods of gastrointestinal decontamination. A summary of the position statement accompanies the description of each procedure.

1. Gastric Lavage

If the patient presents within 60 minutes of ingestion, lavage may be **considered**. Insert an orogastric tube and follow with fluid, usually normal saline. Aspirate back the fluid in an attempt to remove any toxicant. If the patient is neurologically impaired, airway protection with a cuffed endotracheal tube is indicated prior to gastric lavage.

Lavage performed more than 60 minutes after ingestion has not proven to be beneficial and runs the risk of inducing bleeding, perforation, or scarring due to additional trauma to already traumatized tissues. It is almost always necessary first to control seizures before attempting gastric lavage or any other method of GI decontamination.

Studies of poison recovery have been performed mainly with solid material such as pills. There are no controlled studies of pesticide recovery by these methods. Reported recovery of material at 60 minutes in several studies was 8%-32%.[1,2] There is further evidence that lavage may propel the material into the small bowel, thus increasing absorption.[3]

Note on Specific Pesticides: Lavage is contraindicated in hydrocarbon ingestion, a common vehicle in many pesticide formulations.

Position Statement: Gastric lavage should not be routinely used in the management of poisons. Lavage is indicated only when a patient has ingested a potentially life-threatening amount of poison and the procedure can be done within 60 minutes of ingestion. Even then, clinical benefit has not been confirmed in controlled studies.[4]

2. Catharsis

Sorbitol and magnesium citrate are commonly used cathartic agents. Because magnesium citrate has not been studied as much, its use is not described here. Sorbitol is often included in charcoal formulations. It will increase gut motility to improve excretion of the charcoal-poison complex. The dosage of sorbitol is 1-2 g/kg as a one-time dose. Repeat doses of cathartics may result in fluid and electrolyte imbalances, particularly in children, and are therefore not recommended. Sorbitol is formulated in 70% and 35% solutions and usually packaged in 100 mL bottles. The gram dosage of sorbitol in a 100 mL bottle can be calculated by multiplying 100 (mL) x 0.7 (for 70% solution) x 1.285 g sorbitol/mL. Therefore the dose in mL is as follows:

Dosage of Sorbitol:

- *Adults:* 70% sorbitol, 1-2 mL/kg.

- *Children:* 35% sorbitol, 1.5-2.3 mL/kg (maximum dosage: 50 g).

Note on Specific Pesticides: Significant poisoning with organophosphates, carbamates, and arsenicals generally results in a profuse diarrhea. Poisoning with diquat and to a lesser extent paraquat results in an ileus. The use of sorbitol is not recommended in any of the above pesticide poisonings.

Position Statement: The administration of a cathartic alone has no role in the management of the poisoned patient. There are no definite indications for the use of cathartics in the management of the poisoned patient. Data are conflicting with regard to use in combination with activated charcoal, and its routine use is not endorsed. If a cathartic is used, it should be as a single dose in order to minimize adverse effects. There are numerous contraindications, including absent bowel sounds, abdominal trauma or surgery, or intestinal perforation or obstruction. It is also contraindicated in volume depletion, hypotension, electrolyte imbalance, or the ingestion of a corrosive substance.[5]

3. Activated Charcoal Adsorption

Activated charcoal is an effective absorbent for many poisonings. Volunteer studies suggest that it will reduce the amount of poison absorbed if given within 60 minutes.[6] There are insufficient data to support or exclude its use if time from ingestion is prolonged, although some poisons that are less soluble may be adsorbed beyond 60 minutes. Clinical trials with charcoal have been done with poisons other than pesticides. There is some evidence that paraquat is well adsorbed by activated charcoal.[7,8] Charcoal has been anecdotally successful with other pesticides.

> **Dosage of Activated Charcoal:**
>
> - *Adults and children over 12 years:* 25–100 g in 300–800 mL water.
>
> - *Children under 12 years:* 25–50 g per dose.
>
> - *Infants and toddlers under 20 kg:* 1 g per kg body weight.

Many activated charcoal formulations come premixed with sorbitol. Avoid giving more than one dose of sorbitol as a cathartic in infants and children due to the risk of rapid shifts of intravascular fluid.

Encourage the victim to swallow the adsorbent even though spontaneous vomiting continues. Antiemetic therapy may help control vomiting in adults or older children. As an alternative, activated charcoal may be administered through an orogastric tube or diluted with water and administered slowly through a nasogastric tube. Repeated administration of charcoal or other absorbent every 2–4 hours may be beneficial in both children and adults, but use of a cathartic such as sorbitol should be avoided after the first dose. Repeated doses of activated charcoal should not be administered if the gut is atonic. The use of charcoal without airway protection is contraindicated in the neurologically impaired patient.

Note on Specific Pesticides: The use of charcoal without airway protection should be used with caution in poisons such as organophosphates, carbamates, and organochlorines if they are prepared in a hydrocarbon solution.

Position Statement: Single-dose activated charcoal should not be used routinely in the management of poisoned patients. Charcoal appears to be most effective within 60 minutes of ingestion and may be considered for use for this time period. Although it may be considered 60 minutes after ingestion, there is insufficient evidence to support or deny its use for this time period. Despite improved binding of poisons within 60 minutes, only one study exists[9] to suggest that there is improved clinical outcome. Activated charcoal is contraindicated in an unprotected airway, a GI tract not anatomically intact, and when charcoal therapy may increase the risk of **aspiration** of a hydrocarbon-based pesticide.[6]

4. Syrup of Ipecac

Ipecac has been used as an emetic since the 1950s. In a pediatric study, administration of ipecac resulted in vomiting within 30 minutes in 88% of children.[10] However, in light of the recent review of the clinical effectiveness of ipecac, it is **no longer recommended for routine use** in most poisonings. Most clinical trials involve the use of pill form ingestants such as aspirin,[2,11] acetaminophen,[12] ampicillin,[1] and multiple types of tablets.[13] No clinical trials have been done with pesticides. In 1996, more than 2 million human exposures to a poisonous substances were reported to American poison centers. Ipecac was recommended for decontamination in only 1.8% of all exposures.[14]

> ### Dosage of Syrup of Ipecac:
>
> - *Adolescents and adults:* 15-30 mL followed immediately with 240 mL of water.
>
> - *Children 1-12 years:* 15 mL preceded or followed by 120 to 240 mL of water.
>
> - *Infants 6 months to 12 months:* 5-10 mL preceded or followed by 120 to 240 mL of water.
>
> Dose may be repeated in all age groups if emesis does not occur within 20-30 minutes.

Position Statement: Ipecac syrup should not be administered routinely in poisoned patients. If ipecac is used, it should be administered within 60 minutes of the ingestion. Even then, clinical studies have demonstrated no benefit from its use. It should be considered only in an alert conscious patient who has ingested a potentially toxic ingestion. Contraindications to its use include the following: patients with diminished airway protective reflexes, the ingestion of hydrocarbons with a high aspiration potential, the ingestion of a corrosive substance, or the ingestion of a substance in which advanced life support may be necessary within the next 60 minutes.[15]

5. Seizures

Lorazepam is increasingly being recognized as the drug of choice for status epilepticus, although there are few reports of its use with certain pesticides. One must be prepared to assist ventilation with lorazepam and any other medication used to control seizures. See dosage table on next page.

For organochlorine compounds, use of lorazepam has not been reported in the literature. Diazepam is often used for this, and is still used in other pesticide poisonings.

> ### Dosage of Diazepam:
>
> - *Adults:* 5-10 mg IV and repeat every 5-10 minutes to maximum of 30 mg.
>
> - *Children:* 0.2-0.5 mg/kg IV every 5 minutes to maximum of 10 mg in children over 5 years and 5 mg in children under 5 years.

> **Dosage of Lorazepam:**
>
> - *Adults:* 2–4 mg/dose given IV over 2–5 minutes. Repeat if necessary to a maximum of 8 mg in a 12 hour period.
>
> - *Adolescents:* Same as adult dose, except maximum dose is 4 mg.
>
> - *Children under 12 years:* 0.05–0.10 mg/kg IV over 2–5 minutes. Repeat if necessary .05 mg/kg 10–15 minutes after first dose, with a maximum dose of 4 mg.
>
> **Caution:** Be prepared to assist pulmonary ventilation mechanically if respiration is depressed, to intubate the trachea if laryngospasm occurs, and to counteract hypotensive reactions.

Phenobarbital is an additional treatment option for seizure control. Dosage for **infants, children, and adults** is **15–20 mg/kg** as an IV loading dose. An additional 5 mg/kg IV may be given every 15–30 minutes to a maximum of 30 mg/kg. The drug should be pushed no faster than 1 mg/kg/minute.

For seizure management, most patients respond well to usual management consisting of benzodiazepines, or phenytoin and phenobarbital.

References

1. Tenenbein M, Cohen S, and Sitar DS. Efficacy of ipecac-induced emesis, orogastric lavage, and activated charcoal for acute drug overdose. *Ann Emerg Med* 1987;16:838-41.

2. Danel V, Henry JA, and Glucksman E. Activated charcoal, emesis, and gastric lavage in aspirin overdose. *Br Med J* 1988;296:1507.

3. Saetta JP, March S, Gaunt ME, et al. Gastric emptying procedures in the self-poisoned patient: Are we forcing gastric content beyond the pylorus? *J R Soc Med* 1991;84:274-6.

4. American Academy of Clinical Toxicology, European Association of Poisons Centres and Clinical Toxicologists. Position statement: Gastric lavage. *J Toxicol Clin Toxicol* 1997;35:711-9.

5. American Academy of Clinical Toxicology, European Association of Poisons Centres and Clinical Toxicologists. Position statement: Cathartics. *J Toxicol Clin Toxicol* 1997;35:743-52.

6. American Academy of Clinical Toxicology, European Association of Poisons Centres and Clinical Toxicologists. Position statement: Single-dose activated charcoal. *J Toxicol Clin Toxicol* 1997;35:721-41.

7. Gaudreault P, Friedman PA, and Lovejoy FH Jr. Efficacy of activated charcoal and magnesium citrate in the treatment of oral paraquat intoxication. *Ann Emerg Med* 1985;14:123-5.

8. Terada H, Miyoshi T, Imaki M, et al. Studies on in vitro paraquat and diquat removal by activated carbon. *J Exp Med* 1994;41:31-40.

9. Merigian KS, Woodward M, Hedges JR, et al. Prospective evaluation of gastric emptying in the self-poisoned patient. *Am J Emerg Med* 1990;8:479-83.

10. Robertson W. Syrup of ipecac: A slow or fast emetic? *AJDC* 1962;103:136-9.

11. Curtis RA, Barone J, and Giacona N. Efficacy of ipecac and activated charcoal/cathartic. *Arch Intern Med* 1984;144:48-52.

12. McNamara RM, Aaron CK, Gemborys M, et al. Efficacy of charcoal cathartic versus ipecac in reducing serum acetaminophen in a simulated overdose. *Ann Emerg Med* 1989;18:934-8.

13. Neuvonen PJ, Vartiainen M, and Tokola O. Comparison of activated charcoal and ipecac syrup in prevention of drug absorption. *Eur J Clin Pharmacol* 1983;24:557-62.

14. Litovitz RL, Smilkstein M, Felberg L, et al. 1996 Annual Report of the American Association of Poison Control Centers Toxic Exposure Surveillance System. *Am J Emerg Med* 1997;15:447-500.

15. American Academy of Clinical Toxicology, European Association of Poisons Centres and Clinical Toxicologists. Position statement: Ipecac syrup. *J Toxicol Clin Toxicol* 1997;35:699-709.

CHAPTER 3

Environmental and Occupational History

Pesticide poisonings may go unrecognized because of the failure to take a proper exposure history. This chapter is intended to remedy this often overlooked area by providing basic tools for taking a complete exposure history. In some situations where exposures are complex or multiple and/or symptoms atypical, it is important to consider consultation with clinical toxicologists or specialists in environmental and occupational medicine. Local Poison Control Centers should also be considered when there are questions about diagnosis and treatment.

Although this manual deals primarily with pesticide-related diseases and injury, the approach to identifying exposures is similar regardless of the specific hazard involved. It is important to ascertain whether other non-pesticide exposures are involved because of potential interactions between these hazards and the pesticide of interest (e.g., pesticide intoxication and heat stress in agricultural field workers). Thus, the following section on pesticide exposures should be seen in the context of an overall exposure assessment.

Most pesticide-related diseases have clinical presentations that are similar to common medical conditions and display nonspecific symptoms and physical signs. Knowledge of a patient's exposure to occupational and environmental factors is important for diagnostic, therapeutic, rehabilitative and public health purposes. Thus, it is essential to obtain an adequate history of any environmental or occupational exposure which could cause disease or exacerbate an existing medical condition.

In addition to the appropriate patient history-taking, one must also consider any other persons that may be similarly exposed in the home, work or community environment. Each environmental or occupational disease identified should be considered a potential sentinel health event which may require follow-up activities to identify the exposure source and any additional cases. By identifying and eliminating the exposure source, one can prevent continued exposure to the initial patient and any other individuals involved.

Patients with these types of diseases may be seen by health care providers that are not familiar with these conditions. If an appropriate history is obtained and there appears to be a suspect environmental or occupational exposure, the health care provider can obtain consultation with specialists (e.g., industrial hygienists, toxicologists, medical specialists, etc.) in the field of environmental and occupational health. For the more severe sentinel health events and those that involve numerous exposed individuals, additional assistance can be obtained by contacting the state health department, state regulatory agency (e.g., the agriculture department in the case of pesticide illness and injury), or other related organizations (see list at end of chapter). Furthermore, some states require reporting of certain environmental and occupational conditions (e.g., pesticide case reporting in Arizona, California, Florida, Oregon, Texas, and Washington).

This chapter reviews the types of questions to be asked in taking an occupational and environmental history (for both adult and pediatric patients), discusses legal, ethical, and public health considerations, and lists information resources.

Taking an Exposure History

Given the time constraints of most health care providers, a few screening questions are likely to be preferable to a lengthy questionnaire in identifying occupational or environmental hazards. The screening questions below could be incorporated into an existing general health questionnaire or routine patient interview.

SCREENING QUESTIONS FOR OCCUPATIONAL AND ENVIRONMENTAL EXPOSURES*

For an adult patient:
After establishing the chief complaint and history of the presenting illness:

- What kind of work do you do?
- *(if unemployed)* Do you think your health problems are related to your home or other location?
- *(if employed)* Do you think your health problems are related to your work? Are your symptoms better or worse when you are at home or at work?
- Are you now or have you previously been exposed to pesticides, solvents, or other chemicals, dusts, fumes, radiation, or loud noise?

For a pediatric patient (questions asked of parent or guardian):

- Do you think the patient's health problems are related to the home, daycare, school, or other location?
- Has there been any exposure to pesticides, solvents or other chemicals, dusts, fumes, radiation, or loud noise?
- What kind of work do the parents or other household members engage in?

If the clinical presentation or initial medical history suggests a potential occupational or environmental exposure, a detailed exposure interview is needed. An extensive exposure history provides a more complete picture of pertinent exposure factors and can take up to an hour. The detailed interview includes questions on occupational exposure, environmental exposure, symptoms and medical conditions, and non-occupational exposure potentially related to illness or injury. Although the focus is on pesticide exposures and related health effects, concurrent non–pesticide exposures need to be considered in the over-all patient health assessment. Questions typical of a detailed interview are listed on the next several pages, preceded by special concerns in addressing exposures of children and agricultural workers. For further details on taking a history for all types of occupational and environmental hazards, consult the ATSDR mono-graph entitled "Taking an Exposure History"[1] or a general occupational and environmental medicine reference text.[2]

Special Patient Populations

Children

In comparison to adults, children may be at greater risk from pesticide exposures due to growth and developmental factors. Consideration of fetal, infant, toddler or child characteristics is helpful in an exposure evaluation: physical location, breathing zones, oxygen consumption, food consumption, types of foods consumed and normal behavioral development.[3] Furthermore, transpla-cental absorption and breast milk may pose additional routes of exposure. Al-though environmental (and, at times, occupational) exposure to pesticides is the focus of this chapter, the most significant hazard for children is uninten-tional ingestion.[4] Thus, it is very important to ask about pesticides used and stored in the home, day care facility, school, and play areas.

Agricultural Workers

Data from California's mandatory pesticide poisoning reporting system would imply an annual national estimate of 10,000–20,000 cases of farmworker poison-ing.[5] However, it is believed that these figures still represent serious underreporting due to the lack of medical access for many farmworkers and misdiagnosis by some clinicians. For these high-risk patients, the exposure history should include specific questions about the agricultural work being done. For example:

- Are pesticides being used at home or work?
- Were the fields wet when you were picking?
- Was any spraying going on while you were working in the fields?
- Do you get sick during or after working in the fields?

The use of pesticides in the residence and taking home agricultural pesticides or contaminated work clothes that are not properly separated from other clothes may pose hazards for other household members as well.

Obtaining Additional Pesticide Information

In addition to the patient history, it is often helpful to obtain further infor-mation on suspect pesticide products. Two documents are useful starting points

DETAILED INTERVIEW FOR OCCUPATIONAL AND ENVIRONMENTAL EXPOSURES

(Questions marked in bold type are especially important for a pesticide exposure history)

(1) Adult Patient

OCCUPATIONAL EXPOSURE

- **What is your occupation?** (If unemployed, go to next section)
- **How long have you been doing this job?**
- **Describe your work and what hazards you are exposed to (e.g., pesticides,** solvents or other chemicals, dust, fumes, metals, fibers, radiation, biologic agents, noise, heat, cold, vibration)
- **Under what circumstances do you use protective equipment? (e.g., work clothes, safety glasses, respirator, gloves,** and hearing protection)
- **Do you smoke or eat at the worksite?**
- **List previous jobs in chronological order, include full and part-time, temporary, second jobs, summer jobs, and military experience.** *(Because this question can take a long time to answer, one option is to ask the patient to fill out a form with this question on it prior to the formal history taking by the clinician. Another option is to take a shorter history by asking the patient to list only the prior jobs that involved the agents of interest. For example, one could ask for all current and past jobs involving pesticide exposure.)*

ENVIRONMENTAL EXPOSURE HISTORY

- **Are pesticides (e.g., bug or weed killers, flea and tick sprays, collars, powders, or shampoos) used in your home or garden or on your pet?**
- **Do you or any household member have a hobby with exposure to any hazardous materials** (e.g., **pesticides**, paints, ceramics, solvents, metals, glues)?
- **If pesticides are used:**
  - **Is a licensed pesticide applicator involved?**
  - **Are children allowed to play in areas recently treated with pesticides?**
  - **Where are the pesticides stored?**
  - **Is food handled properly (e.g., washing of raw fruits and vegetables)?**
- **Did you ever live near a facility which could have contaminated the surrounding area** (e.g., mine, **plant**, smelter, **dump site**)?
- **Have you ever changed your residence because of a health problem?**
- **Does your drinking water come from a private well, city water supply, and/or grocery store?**
- Do you work on your car?
- Which of the following do you have in your home: air conditioner/purifier, central heating (gas or oil), gas stove, electric stove, fireplace, wood stove, or humidifier?
- Have you recently acquired new furniture or carpet, or remodeled your home?
- Have you weatherized your home recently?
- Approximately what year was your home built?

SYMPTOMS AND MEDICAL CONDITIONS

(If employed)
- **Does the timing of your symptoms have any relationship to your work hours?**
- **Has anyone else at work suffered the same or similar problems?**
- **Does the timing of your symptoms have any relationship to environmental activities listed above?**
- **Has any other household member or nearby neighbor suffered similar health problems?**

NON-OCCUPATIONAL EXPOSURES POTENTIALLY RELATED TO ILLNESS OR INJURY

- **Do you use tobacco?** If yes, in what forms (cigarettes, pipe, cigar, chewing tobacco)? About how many do you smoke or how much tobacco do you use per day? At what age did you start using tobacco? Are there other tobacco smokers in the home?

- **Do you drink alcohol?** How much per day or week? At what age did you start?

- **What medications or drugs are you taking?** *(Include prescription and non-prescription uses)*

- **Has anyone in the family worked with hazardous materials that they might have brought home (e.g., pesticides,** asbestos, lead)? *(If yes, inquire about household members potentially exposed.)*

(2) Pediatric Patient (questions asked of parent or guardian)

OCCUPATIONAL EXPOSURE

- **What is your occupation and that of other household members?** (If no employed individuals, go to next section)

- **Describe your work and what hazards you are exposed to (e.g., pesticides,** solvents or other chemicals, dust, fumes, metals, fibers, radiation, biologic agents, noise, heat, cold, vibration)

ENVIRONMENTAL EXPOSURE HISTORY

- **Are pesticides (e.g., bug or weed killers, flea and tick sprays, collars, powders, or shampoos) used in your home or garden or on your pet?**

- **Do you or any household member have a hobby with exposure to any hazardous materials (e.g., pesticides,** paints, ceramics, solvents, metals, glues**)?**

- **If pesticides are used:**
  - **Is a licensed pesticide applicator involved?**
  - **Are children allowed to play in areas recently treated with pesticides?**
  - **Where are the pesticides stored?**
  - **Is food handled properly (e.g., washing of raw fruits and vegetables)?**

- **Has the patient ever lived near a facility which could have contaminated the surrounding area** (e.g., mine, **plant**, smelter, **dump site**)?

- **Has the patient ever changed residence because of a health problem?**

- **Does the patient's drinking water come from a private well, city water supply, and/or grocery store?**

- Which of the following are in the patient's home: air conditioner/purifier, central heating (gas or oil), gas stove, electric stove, fireplace, wood stove, or humidifier?

- Is there recently acquired new furniture or carpet, or recent home remodeling in the patient's home?

- Has the home been weatherized recently?

- Approximately what year was the home built?

SYMPTOMS AND MEDICAL CONDITIONS

- **Does the timing of symptoms have any relationship to environmental activities listed above?**

- **Has any other household member or nearby neighbor suffered similar health problems?**

NON-OCCUPATIONAL EXPOSURES POTENTIALLY RELATED TO ILLNESS OR INJURY

- **Are there tobacco smokers in the home?** If yes, in what forms (cigarettes, pipe, cigar, chewing tobacco)?

- **What medications or drugs is the patient taking?** *(Include prescription and non-prescription uses)*

- **Has anyone in the family worked with hazardous materials that they might have brought home (e.g., pesticides,** asbestos, lead)? *(If yes, inquire about household members potentially exposed.)*

in the identification and evaluation of the pesticide exposure: the material safety data sheet (MSDS) and the pesticide label.

- **Material Safety Data Sheet (MSDS).** Under OSHA's Hazard Communications Standard (29 CFR 1910.1200), all chemical manufacturers are required to provide an MSDS for each hazardous chemical they produce or import. Employers are required to keep copies of MSDSs and make them available to the workers. The following items are contained in an MSDS:

  - Material identification
  - Ingredients and occupational exposure limits
  - Physical data
  - Fire and explosion data
  - Reactivity data
  - Health hazard data
  - Spill, leak, and disposal procedures
  - Special protection data
  - Special precautions and comments.

  These documents tend to have very limited information on health effects and some of the active ingredients may be omitted due to trade secret considerations. One cannot rely solely on an MSDS in making medical determinations.

- **Pesticide label.** EPA requires that all pesticide products bear labels that provide certain information. This information can help in evaluating pesticide health effects and necessary precautions. The items covered include the following:

  - Product name
  - Manufacturer
  - EPA registration number
  - Active ingredients
  - Precautionary statements:

    i. Human hazard signal words "Danger" (most hazardous), "Warning," and "Caution" (least hazardous)

    ii. Child hazard warning

    iii. Statement of practical treatment (signs and symptoms of poisoning, first aid, antidotes, and note to physicians in the event of a poisoning)

    iv. Hazards to humans and domestic animals

    v. Environmental hazards

    vi. Physical or chemical hazards

- Directions for use
- Name and address of manufacturer
- Net contents
- EPA registration number
- EPA establishment number
- Worker Protection Standard (WPS) designation, including restricted entry interval and personal protection equipment required (see WPS description on page 25).

The EPA registration number is useful when contacting EPA for information or when calling the National Pesticide Telecommunications Network hotline (see page 29). Pesticide labels may differ from one state to another based on area-specific considerations. Also, different formulations of the same active ingredients may result in different label information. The pesticide label lists information only for active ingredients (not for inert components) and rarely contains information on chronic health effects (e.g., cancer and neurologic, reproductive, and respiratory diseases).[6] Although further pesticide information is often needed, these documents should be considered as the first step in identifying and understanding the health effects of a given pesticide.

For the agricultural worker patient, the health care provider has two legal bases — the EPA Worker Protection Standard and USDA regulations under the 1990 Farm Bill — for obtaining from the employer the pesticide product name to which the patient was exposed. When requesting this information, the clinician should keep the patient's name confidential whenever possible.

Assessing the Relationship of Work or Environment to Disease

Because pesticides and other chemical and physical hazards are often associated with nonspecific medical complaints, it is very important to link the review of systems with the timing of suspected exposure to the hazardous agent. The Index of Signs and Symptoms in Section V provides a quick reference to symptoms and medical conditions associated with specific pesticides. Further details on the toxicology, confirmatory tests, and treatment of illnesses related to pesticides are provided in each chapter of this manual. A general understanding of pesticide classes and some of the more common agents is helpful in making a pesticide related disease diagnoses.

In evaluating the association of a given pesticide exposure in the workplace or environment and a clinical condition, key factors to consider are:

- Symptoms and physical signs appropriate for the pesticide being considered

- Co-workers or others in the environment who are ill

- Timing of the problems

- Confirmation of physical exposure to the pesticide

- Environmental monitoring data

- Biomonitoring results

- Biological plausibility of the resulting health effect

- Ruling out non-pesticide exposures or pre-existing illnesses.

A concurrent non-pesticide exposure can either have no health effect, exacerbate an existing pesticide health effect, or solely cause the health effect in a patient. In the more complicated exposure scenarios, assistance should be sought from specialists in occupational and environmental health (see Information Resources on page 27).

Legal, Ethical, and Public Health Considerations

Following are some considerations related to government regulation of pesticides, ethical factors, and public health concerns that health care providers should be aware of in assessing a possible pesticide exposure.

Reporting Requirements

When evaluating a patient with a pesticide-related medical condition, it is important to understand the state-specific reporting requirements for the workers' compensation system (if there has been an occupational exposure) or surveillance system. Reporting a workers' compensation case can have significant implications for the worker being evaluated. If the clinician is not familiar with this system or is uncomfortable evaluating work-related health events, it is important to seek an occupational medicine consultation or make an appropriate referral.

At least six states have surveillance systems within their state health departments that cover both occupational and environmental pesticide poisonings: California, Florida, New York, Oregon, Texas, and Washington. These surveillance systems collect case reports on pesticide-related illness and injury from clinicians and other sources; conduct selected interviews, field investigations, and research projects; and function as a resource for pesticide information within their state. In some states, as noted earlier, pesticide case reporting is legally mandated.

Regulatory Agencies

Since its formation in 1970, EPA has been the lead agency for the regulation of pesticide use under the Federal Insecticide, Fungicide and Rodenticide Act. EPA's mandates include the registration of all pesticides used in the United States, setting restricted entry intervals, specification and approval of label information, and setting acceptable food and water tolerance levels. In addition, EPA works in partnership with state and tribal agencies to implement two field programs — the certification and training program for pesticide applicators and the agricultural worker protection standard — to protect workers and handlers from pesticide exposures. EPA sets national standards for certification of over 1 million private and commercial pesticide applicators.

The authority to enforce EPA regulations is delegated to the states. For example, calls concerning non-compliance with the worker protection standard can typically be made to the state agricultural department. In five states, the department of the environment or other state agency has enforcement authority. Anonymous calls can be made if workers anticipate possible retaliatory action by management. It should be noted that not all state departments of agriculture have similar regulations. In California, for instance, employers are required to obtain medical supervision and biological monitoring of agricultural workers who apply pesticides containing cholinesterase-inhibiting compounds. This requirement is not found in the federal regulations.

Outside the agricultural setting, the Occupational Safety and Health Administration (OSHA) has jurisdiction over workplace exposures. All workers involved in pesticide manufacturing would be covered by OSHA. OSHA sets permissible exposure levels for selected pesticides. Approximately half the states are covered by the federal OSHA; the rest have their own state-plan OSHA. Individual state plans may choose to be more protective in setting their workplace standards. Anonymous calls can also be made to either state-plan or federal OSHA agencies.

For pesticide contamination in water, EPA sets enforceable maximum containment levels. In food and drug-related outbreaks, EPA works jointly with the Food and Drug Administration (FDA) and the U.S. Department of Agriculture (USDA) to monitor and regulate pesticide residues and their metabolites. Tolerance limits are established for many pesticides and their metabolites in raw agricultural commodities.

In evaluating a patient with pesticide exposure, the clinician may need to report a pesticide intoxication to the appropriate health and/or regulatory agency.

Worker Protection Standard

EPA's Worker Protection Standard (WPS) became fully effective in 1995. The intent of the regulation is to eliminate or reduce pesticide exposure, mitigate exposures that occur, and inform agricultural workers about the hazards of pesticides. The WPS applies to two types of workers in the farm, greenhouse, nursery, and forest industries: (1) agricultural pesticide handlers (mixer, loader, applicator, equipment cleaner or repair person, and flagger), and (2) field workers (cultivator or harvester).

The WPS includes requirements that agricultural employers notify workers about pesticide treatments in advance, offer basic pesticide safety training, provide personal protective equipment for direct work with pesticides, and observe restricted entry interval (REI) times. (The REI is a required waiting period before workers can return to areas treated with pesticides.) Of special interest to health care providers, the WPS also requires agricultural employers to:

- Post an emergency medical facility address and phone number in a central location.

- Arrange immediate transport from the agricultural establishment to a medical facility for a pesticide-affected worker.

- Supply the affected worker and medical personnel with product name, EPA registration number, active ingredient, label medical information, a description of how the pesticide was used, and exposure information.

Ethical Considerations

Attempts to investigate an occupational pesticide exposure may call for obtaining further information from the worksite manager or owner. Any contact with the worksite should be taken in consultation with the patient because of the potential for retaliatory actions (such as loss of job or pay cuts). Ideally, a request for a workplace visit or more information about pesticide exposure at the workplace will occur with the patient's agreement. In situations where the health hazard is substantial and many individuals might be affected, a call to a state pesticide surveillance system (if available), agricultural health and safety center (if nearby), can provide the National Institute for Occupational Safety and Health (NIOSH) or state agricultural agency the assistance needed for a disease outbreak investigation.

Similarly, the discovery of pesticide contamination in a residence, school, daycare setting, food product, or other environmental site or product can have public health, financial, and legal consequences for the patient and other individuals (e.g., building owner, school district, food producer). It is prudent to discuss these situations and follow-up options with the patient as well as a knowledgeable environmental health specialist and appropriate state or local agencies.

Public Health Considerations

Health care providers are often the first to identify a sentinel health event that upon further investigation develops into a full-blown disease outbreak. A disease outbreak is defined as a statistically elevated rate of disease among a well-defined population as compared to a standard population. For example, complaints about infertility problems among workers at a dibromochloropropane (DBCP) manufacturing plant in California led to diagnoses of azoospermia (lack of sperm) or oligospermia (decreased sperm count) among a handful of otherwise healthy young men working at the plant.[7] An eventual disease outbreak investigation resulted in the first published report of a male reproductive toxicant in the workplace. At the time, DBCP was used as a nematocide; it has since been banned in the United States.

Disease outbreak investigations are conducted for all kinds of exposures and health events, not only those in the occupational and environmental area. Usually, assistance from government or university experts is needed in the investigation, which may require access to information, expertise, and resources beyond that available to the average clinician. The steps involved in such an investigation and the types of information typically gathered in the preliminary clinical stages are outlined below. The clinician must be aware that an outbreak investigation may be needed when a severe and widespread exposure and disease scenario exists. For more information on disease outbreak investigations, consult the literature.[8, 9]

STEPS IN INVESTIGATING A DISEASE OUTBREAK

- Confirm diagnosis of initial case reports (the "index" cases)
- Identify other unrecognized cases
- Establish a case definition
- Characterize cases by person, place, and time characteristics (e.g., age, race, ethnicity, gender, location within a company or a neighborhood, timeline of exposure and health events)
- Create plot of case incidence by time (an epidemic curve)
- Determine if a dose-response relationship exists (i.e., more severe clinical case presentation for individuals with higher exposures)
- Derive an attack rate and determine if statistical significance is achieved (divide number of incident cases by number of exposed individuals and multiply by 100 to obtain attack rate percentage)

Information Resources

Government Agencies:

EPA Office of Pesticide Programs
Overall pesticide regulation with special programs on agricultural workers and pesticide applicators. Specific programs include the promotion of the reduction of pesticide use, establishment of tolerance levels for food, and investigation of pesticide releases and exposure events.

Address: EPA – Office of Pesticide Programs
                 401 M Street SW (7501C)
                 Washington, DC 20460
Telephone: 703-305-7090
Web site: www.epa.gov/pesticides

EPA – Certification and Worker Protection Branch
Within the Office of Pesticide Programs, the Certification and Worker Protection Branch addresses worker-related pesticide issues and pesticide applicator certification activities. Special emphasis is placed on the adequate training of farm workers, pesticide applicators, and health care providers. Various training

materials in several languages are available.

Address: EPA – OPP
             401 M Street SW (7506C)
             Washington, DC 20460
Telephone: 703-305-7666
Web site: www.epa.gov/pesticides/safety

Occupational Safety and Health Administration (OSHA)

More than 100 million workers and 6.5 million employers are covered under the Occupational Safety and Health Act, which covers workers in pesticide manufacturing as well as other industries. OSHA and its state partners have approximately 2100 inspectors, plus investigators, standards writers, educators, physicians, and other staff in over 200 offices across the country. OSHA sets protective workplace standards, enforces the standards, and offers employers and employees technical assistance and consultation programs. Note that some states have their own OSHA plan.

Address: OSHA – US DOL
             Room N3647
             Constitution Ave NW
             Washington, DC 20210
Telephone: 202-219-8021
Web site: www.osha.gov

Food and Drug Administration (FDA)

Drug and food pesticide issues.

Address: FDA
             National Center for Toxicological Research
             5600 Fishers Lane
             Rockville, MD 20857
Telephone: 301-443-3170
Internet: gopher.nctr.fda.gov

USDA Extension Service

USDA's Extension Service works with its university partners, the state land-grant system, to provide farmers and ranchers information to reduce and prevent agricultural-related work incidents. The Pesticide Applicator Training program trains applicators in the safe use of pesticides and coordinates pesticide-related safety training programs.

Address: USDA
             14th & Independence SW
             Washington, DC 20250
Telephone: 202-720-2791
Web site: www.reeusda.gov

National Center for Environmental Health (NCEH), Centers for Disease Control (CDC)

NCEH provides expertise in environmental pesticide case surveillance and disease outbreak investigations.

Address: NCEH, CDC
             Mailstop F29
             4770 Buford Highway NE
             Atlanta, GA 30341
Tel: 770-488-7030
Web site: www.cdc.gov/nceh/ncehhome.htm

National Institute for Occupational Safety and Health (NIOSH), Centers for Disease Control (CDC)

NIOSH is the federal agency responsible for conducting research on occupational disease and injury. NIOSH may investigate potentially hazardous working conditions upon request, makes recommendations on preventing workplace disease and injury, and provides training to occupational safety and health professionals.

Address: NIOSH
             Humphrey Building, Room 715H
             200 Independence Ave SW
             Washington, DC 20201
Hotline: 1-800-356-4674
Web site: www.cdc.gov/niosh/homepage.html

NIOSH Agricultural Health and Safety Centers

NIOSH has funded eight Agricultural Health and Safety Centers throughout the country which involve clinicians and other health specialists in the area of pesticide-related illness and injury. The NIOSH-supported centers are:

University of California Agricultural Health and Safety Center
Old Davis Road
University of California
Davis, CA 95616
Tel: 916-752-4050

High Plains Intermountain Center for Agricultural Health and Safety
Colorado State University
Fort Collins, CO 80523
Tel: 970-491-6152

Great Plains Center for Agricultural Health
University of Iowa
Iowa City, IA 52242
Tel: 319-335-4415

Southeast Center for Agricultural Health and Injury Prevention
University of Kentucky
Department of Preventive Medicine
Lexington, KY 40536
Tel: 606-323-6836

Northeast Center for Agricultural and Occupational Health
One Atwell Road
Cooperstown, NY 13326
Tel: 607-547-6023

Southwest Center for Agricultural Health, Injury and Education
University of Texas
Health Center at Tyler
PO Box 2003
Tyler, TX 75710
Tel: 903-877-5896

Pacific Northwest Agricultural Safety and Health Center
University of Washington
Department of Environmental Health
Seattle, WA 98195
Tel: 206-543-0916

Midwest Center for Agricultural Research, Education and Disease and Injury Prevention
National Farm Medicine Center
Marshfield, WI 54449-5790
Tel: 715-389-3415

Non-Governmental Organizations:

National Pesticide Telecommunications Network

The National Pesticide Telecommunications Network (NPTN) is based at Oregon State University and is cooperatively sponsored by the University and EPA. NPTN serves as a source of objective, science-based pesticide information on a wide range of pesticide-related topics, such as recognition and management of pesticide poisonings, safety information, health and environmental effects, referrals for investigation of pesticide incidents and emergency treatment for both humans and animals, and cleanup and disposal procedures.

A toll-free telephone service provides pesticide information to callers in the continental United States, Puerto Rico, and the Virgin Islands. Additionally, pesticide questions and comments can be sent to an e-mail address. The Web site has links to other sites and databases for further information.

NPTN hotline: 1-800-858-7378
Hours of operation: 9:30 am – 7:30 pm E.S.T. daily except holidays
Web site: http://ace.orst.edu/info/nptn/
E-mail address: nptn@ace.orst.edu

Farmworker Justice Fund

The Farmworker Justice Fund can provide an appropriate referral to a network of legal services and nonprofit groups which represent farmworkers for free.

Address: Farmworker Justice Fund
                1111 19th Street, NW, Suite 1000
                Washington, DC 20036
Telephone: 202-776-1757
E-mail address: fjf@nclr.org

American Farm Bureau Federation

The AFBF is the nation's largest general farm organization. Information on how to contact individual state-based farm bureaus is available on their Web site.

Web site: www.fb.com

Association of Occupational and Environmental Clinics (AOEC)

This association is a network of 63 clinics representing more than 250 specialists.

Address: AOEC
               1010 Vermont Ave, NW, Suite 513
               Washington, DC 20005
Telephone: 202-347-4976
Web site: http://152.3.65.120/oem/aoec.htm

Poison Control Centers

For a list of state and regional poison control centers, or the nearest location, consult the NPTN Web site (http://ace.orst.edu/info/nptn).

Pesticide Information Databases:

Extension Toxicology Network (EXTOXNET)

http://ace.ace.orst.edu/info/extoxnet

The Extension Service's Toxicology Network, EXTOXNET, provides science-based information about pesticides to health care providers treating pesticide-related health concerns. Pesticide toxicological information is developed cooperatively by the University of California-Davis, Oregon State University, Michigan State University, Cornell University, and the University of Idaho.

IRIS

www.epa.gov/ngispgm3/iris

The Integrated Risk Information System – IRIS – is an electronic database, maintained by EPA, on human health effects that may result from exposure to various chemicals in the environment. IRIS is intended for those without extensive training in toxicology, but with some knowledge of health sciences. It provides hazard identification and dose-response assessment information. Combined with specific exposure information, the data in IRIS can be used for characterization of the public health risks of a chemical in a particular situation that can lead to a risk management decision designed to protect public health. Extensive supporting documentation available online.

Agency for Toxic Substances and Disease Registry

http://atsdr1.atsdr.cdc.gov:8080/toxfaq.html

ATSDR (part of the Department of Human Health and Services) publishes fact sheets and other information on pesticides and other toxic substances.

California Pesticide Databases

http://www.cdpr.ca.gov/docs/database/database.htm

Includes Pesticidal Chemical Ingredients Queries, links to EPA's Officeof Pesticide Programs chemical dictionary, Product/Label Database Queries (updated nightly), a current listing of California's Section 18 Emergency Exemptions, and more.

References

1. Frank A and Balk S. ATSDR Case Studies in Environmental Medicine #26, Taking an Exposure History. Atlanta: Agency for Toxic Substances and Disease Registry, Oct. 1992.

2. LaDou J. Approach to the diagnosis of occupational illness. In: LaDou J (ed). Occupational and Environmental Medicine, 2nd ed. Stamford, CT: Appleton and Lange, 1997.

3. Bearer C. Chapter 10: Pediatric developmental toxicology. In: Brooks SM, Gochfield M, Herzstein J, et al. Environmental Medicine. St. Louis, MO: Mosby Yearbook, 1995, pp. 115-28.

4. Jackson RJ. Chapter 31: Hazards of pesticides to children. Ibid, pp. 377-82.

5. Blondell JM. Epidemiology of pesticide poisonings in the United States, with special reference to occupational cases. In: Keifer MC (ed). Human Health Effects of Pesticides, Occupational Medicine: State of the Art Reviews, Philadelphia: Hanley & Belfus, Inc., 1997.

6. Keifer MC (ed). Ibid.

7. Osorio, AM. Chapter 26: Male reproductive toxicology. In: LaDou J (ed), op. cit.

8. Brooks SM, Gochfield M, Herzstein J, et al. Environmental Medicine. St. Louis, MO: Mosby Yearbook, 1995.

9. Steenland K. Case Studies in Occupational Epidemiology. New York: Oxford University Press, 1993.

Section II

INSECTICIDES

CHAPTER 4

Organophosphate Insecticides

HIGHLIGHTS

- Acts through phosphorylation of the acetylcholinesterase enzyme at nerve endings
- Absorbed by inhalation, ingestion, and skin penetration
- Muscarinic, nicotinic & CNS effects

Signs and Symptoms:

- Headache, hypersecretion, muscle twitching, nausea, diarrhea
- Respiratory depression, seizures, loss of consciousness
- Miosis is often a helpful diagnostic sign

Treatment:

- Clear airway, improve tissue oxygenation
- Administer atropine sulfate intravenously
- Pralidoxime may be indicated
- Proceed concurrently with decontamination

Contraindicated:

- Morphine, succinylcholine, theophylline, phenothiazines, reserpine

Since the removal of organochlorine insecticides from use, organophosphate insecticides have become the most widely used insecticides available today. More than forty of them are currently registered for use and all run the risk of acute and subacute toxicity. Organophosphates are used in agriculture, in the home, in gardens, and in veterinary practice. All apparently share a common mechanism of cholinesterase inhibition and can cause similar symptoms. Because they share this mechanism, exposure to the same organophosphate by multiple routes or to multiple organophosphates by multiple routes can lead to serious additive toxicity. It is important to understand, however, that there is a wide range of toxicity in these agents and wide variation in cutaneous absorption, making specific identification and management quite important.

Toxicology

Organophosphates poison insects and mammals primarily by phosphorylation of the acetylcholinesterase enzyme (AChE) at nerve endings. The result is a loss of available AChE so that the effector organ becomes overstimulated by the excess acetylcholine (ACh, the impulse-transmitting substance) in the nerve ending. The enzyme is critical to normal control of nerve impulse transmission from nerve fibers to smooth and skeletal muscle cells, glandular cells, and autonomic ganglia, as well as within the central nervous system (CNS). Some critical proportion of the tissue enzyme mass must be inactivated by phosphorylation before symptoms and signs of poisoning become manifest.

At sufficient dosage, loss of enzyme function allows accumulation of ACh peripherally at cholinergic neuroeffector junctions (muscarinic effects), skeletal nerve-muscle junctions, and autonomic ganglia (nicotinic effects), as well as centrally. At cholinergic nerve junctions with smooth muscle and gland cells, high ACh concentration causes muscle contraction and secretion, respectively. At skeletal muscle junctions, excess ACh may be excitatory (cause muscle twitching), but may also weaken or paralyze the cell by depolarizing the end-plate. In the CNS, high ACh concentrations cause sensory and behavioral disturbances, incoordination, depressed motor function, and respiratory depression. Increased pulmonary secretions coupled with respiratory failure are the usual causes of death from organophosphate poisoning. Recovery depends ultimately on generation of new enzyme in all critical tissues.

COMMERCIAL PRODUCTS

acephate
  Orthene
azinphos-methyl+
  Gusathion
  Guthion
bensulide
  Betasan
  Lescosan
bomyl+
  Swat
bromophos
  Nexion
bromophos-ethyl
  Nexagan
cadusafos
  Apache
  Ebufos
  Rugby
carbophenothion+
  Trithion
chlorethoxyfos
  Fortress
chlorfenvinphos
  Apachlor
  Birlane
chlormephos+
  Dotan
chlorphoxim
  Baythion-C
chlorpyrifos
  Brodan
  Dursban
  Lorsban
chlorthiophos+
  Celathion
coumaphos+
  Asuntol
  Co-Ral
crotoxyphos
  Ciodrin
  Cypona
crufomate
  Ruelene
cyanofenphos+
  Surecide
cyanophos
  Cyanox
cythioate
  Cyflee
  Proban
DEF
  De-Green
  E-Z-Off D
demeton+
  systox
demeton-S-methyl
  Duratox
  Metasystoxl
dialifor+
  Torak
diazinon
dichlorofenthion

VC-13 Nemacide
dichlorvos
  DDVP
  Vapona
dicrotophos+
  Bidrin
dimefos+
  Hanane
  Pestox XIV
dimethoate
  Cygon
  DeFend
dioxathion+
  Delnav
disulfoton+
  Disyston
ditalimfos
  edifenphos
endothion+
EPBP
  S-Seven
EPN+
ethion
  Ethanox
ethoprop
  Mocap
ethyl parathion+
  E605
  Parathion
  thiophos
etrimfos
  Ekamet
famphur+
  Bash
  Bo-Ana
  Famfos
fenamiphos+
  Nemacur
fenitrothion
  Accothion
  Agrothion
  Sumithion
fenophosphon+
  Agritox
  trichloronate
fensulfothion+
  Dasanit
fenthion
  Baytex
  Entex
  Tiguvon
fonofos+
  Dyfonate
  N-2790
formothion
  Anthio
fosthietan+
  Nem-A-Tak
heptenophos
  Hostaquick
hiometon
  Ekatin

hosalone
  Zolone
IBP
  Kitazin
iodofenphos
  Nuvanol-N
isazofos
  Brace
  Miral
  Triumph
isofenphos+
  Amaze
  Oftanol
isoxathion
  E-48
  Karphos
leptophos
  Phosvel
malathion
  Cythion
mephosfolan+
  Cytrolane
merphos
  Easy off-D
  Folex
methamidophos+
  Monitor
methidathion+
  Supracide
  Ultracide
methyl parathion+
  E 601
  Penncap-M
methyl trithion
mevinphos+
  Duraphos
  Phosdrin
mipafox+
  Isopestox
  Pestox XV
monocrotophos+
  Azodrin
naled
  Dibrom
oxydemeton-methyl
  Metasystox-R
oxydeprofos
  Metasystox-S
phencapton
  G 28029
phenthoate
  dimephenthoate
  Phenthoate
phorate+
  Rampart
  Thimet
phosalone
  Azofene
  Zolone
phosfolan+
  Cylan
  Cyolane

phosmet
  Imidan
  Prolate
phosphamidon+
  Dimecron
phostebupirim
  Aztec
phoxim
  Baython
pirimiphos-ethyl
  Primicid
pirimiphos-methyl
  Actellic
profenofos
  Curacron
propetamphos
  Safrotin
propyl thiopyro-
  phosphate+
  Aspon
prothoate
  Fac
pyrazophos
  Afugan
  Curamil
pyridaphenthion
  Ofunack
quinalphos
  Bayrusil
ronnel
  Fenchlorphos
  Korlan
schradan+
  OMPA
sulfotep+
  Bladafum
  Dithione
  Thiotepp
sulprofos
  Bolstar
  Helothion
temephos
  Abate
  Abathion
terbufos
  Contraven
  Counter
tetrachlorvinphos
  Gardona
  Rabon
tetraethyl pyrophos-
  phate+
  TEPP
triazophos
  Hostathion
trichlorfon
  Dipterex
  Dylox
  Neguvon
  Proxol

+ Indicates high toxicity. Highly toxic organophosphates have listed oral LD_{50} values (rat) less than or equal to 50 mg/kg body weight. Most other organophosphates included in this table are considered moderately toxic, with LD_{50} values in excess of 50 mg/kg and less than 500 mg/kg.

Organophosphates are efficiently absorbed by inhalation, ingestion, and skin penetration. There is considerable variation in the relative absorption by these various routes. For instance, the oral LD_{50} of parathion in rats is between 3–8 mg/kg, which is quite toxic,[1,2] and essentially equivalent to dermal absorption with an LD_{50} of 8 mg/kg.[2] On the other hand, the toxicity of **phosalone** is much lower from the dermal route than the oral route, with rat LD_{50}s of 1500 mg/kg and 120 mg/kg, respectively.[2] In general, the highly toxic agents are more likely to have high-order dermal toxicity than the moderately toxic agents.

Chemical Classes: To some degree, the occurrence of poisoning depends on the rate at which the pesticide is absorbed. Breakdown occurs chiefly by hydrolysis in the liver; rates of hydrolysis vary widely from one compound to another. In the case of certain organophosphates whose breakdown is relatively slow, significant temporary storage in body fat may occur. Some organophosphates such as diazinon and methyl parathion have significant lipid solubility, allowing fat storage with delayed toxicity due to late release.[3] Delayed toxicity may also occur atypically with other organophosphates, specifically dichlorofenthion and demeton-methyl.[4] Many organothiophosphates readily undergo conversion from thions (P=S) to oxons (P=O). Conversion occurs in the environment under the influence of oxygen and light, and in the body, chiefly by the action of liver microsomes. Oxons are much more toxic than thions, but oxons break down more readily. Ultimately, both thions and oxons are hydrolyzed at the ester linkage, yielding alkyl phosphates and leaving groups, both of which are of relatively low toxicity. They are either excreted or further transformed in the body before excretion.

The distinction between the different chemical classes becomes important when the physician interprets tests from reference laboratories. This can be especially important when the lab analyzes for the parent compound (i.e., chlorpyrifos in its thiophosphate form) instead of the metabolite form (chlorpyrifos will be completely metabolized to the oxon after the first pass through the liver).

Within one or two days of initial organophosphate binding to AChE, some phosphorylated acetylcholinesterase enzyme can be de-phosphorylated (reactivated) by the oxime antidote pralidoxime. As time progresses, the enzyme-phosphoryl bond is strengthened by loss of one alkyl group from the phosphoryl adduct, a process called aging. Pralidoxime reactivation is therefore no longer possible after a couple of days,[5] although in some cases, improvement has still been seen with pralidoxime administration days after exposure.[6]

OPIDN: Rarely, certain organophosphates have caused a different kind of neurotoxicity consisting of damage to the afferent fibers of peripheral and central nerves and associated with inhibition of "neuropathy target esterase" (NTE). This delayed syndrome has been termed organophosphate-induced delayed neuropathy (OPIDN), and is manifested chiefly by weakness or paralysis and paresthesia of the extremities.[7] OPIDN predominantly affects the legs and may persist for weeks to years. These rare occurrences have been found shortly after an acute and often massive exposure, but in some cases, symptoms have persisted for months to years. Only a few of the many organophosphates used as pesticides have been implicated as causes of delayed neuropathy in humans. EPA guidelines require that organophosphate and carbamate compounds which are candidate pesticides be tested in susceptible animal species for this neurotoxic property.

Three epidemiologic studies with an exposed group and a control group also suggest that a proportion of patients acutely poisoned from any organophosphate can experience some long-term neuropsychiatric sequelae. The findings show significantly worse performance on a battery of neurobehavioral tests, including memory, concentration, and mood, and compound-specific peripheral neuropathy in some cases. These findings are subtle and may sometimes be picked up only on neuropsychologic testing rather than on a neurologic exam.[8-10] Follow-ups of case series have occasionally found some individuals reporting persistent headaches, blurred vision, muscle weakness, depression, memory and concentration problems, irritability, and/or development of intolerance to selected chemical odors.[11-15]

Intermediate Syndrome: In addition to acute poisoning episodes and OPIDN, an intermediate syndrome has been described. This syndrome occurs after resolution of the acute cholinergic crisis, generally 24-96 hours after exposure. It is characterized by acute respiratory paresis and muscular weakness, primarily in the facial, neck, and proximal limb muscles. In addition, it is often accompanied by cranial nerve palsies and depressed tendon reflexes. Like OPIDN, this syndrome lacks muscarinic symptomatology, and appears to result from a combined pre- and post-synaptic dysfunction of neuromuscular transmission. Symptoms do not respond well to atropine and oximes; therefore treatment is mainly supportive.[16,17] The most common compounds involved in this syndrome are methyl parathion, fenthion, and dimethoate, although one case with ethyl parathion was also observed.[17]

Other specific properties of individual organophosphates may render them more hazardous than basic toxicity data suggest. By-products can develop in long-stored malathion which strongly inhibit the hepatic enzymes operative in malathion degradation, thus enhancing its toxicity. Certain organophosphates are exceptionally prone to storage in fat tissue, prolonging the need for antidote for several days as stored pesticide is released back into the circulation. Animal studies have demonstrated potentiation of effect when two or more organophosphates are absorbed simultaneously; enzymes critical to the degradation of one are inhibited by the other. Animal studies have also demonstrated a protective effect from phenobarbital which induces hepatic degradation of the pesticide.[1] Degradation of some compounds to a trimethyl phosphate can cause restrictive lung disease.[18]

Signs and Symptoms of Poisoning

Symptoms of acute organophosphate poisoning develop during or after exposure, within minutes to hours, depending on the method of contact. Exposure by inhalation results in the fastest appearance of toxic symptoms, followed by the gastrointestinal route and finally the dermal route. All signs and symptoms are cholinergic in nature and affect muscarinic, nicotinic, and central nervous system receptors.[5] The critical symptoms in management are the respiratory symptoms. Sufficient muscular fasciculations and weakness are often observed as to require respiratory support; respiratory arrest can occur suddenly. Likewise, bronchorrhea and bronchospasm may often impede efforts at adequate oxygenation of the patient.

Bronchospasm and bronchorrhea can occur, producing tightness in the chest, wheezing, productive cough, and pulmonary edema. A life threatening severity of poisoning is signified by loss of consciousness, incontinence, convulsions, and respiratory depression. The primary cause of death is respiratory failure, and there usually is a secondary cardiovascular component. The classic cardiovascular sign is bradycardia which can progress to sinus arrest. However, this may be superseded by tachycardia and hypertension from nicotinic (sympathetic ganglia) stimulation.[19] Toxic myocardiopathy has been a prominent feature of some severe organophosphate poisonings.

Some of the most commonly reported early symptoms include headache, nausea, dizziness, and hypersecretion, the latter of which is manifested by sweating, salivation, lacrimation, and rhinorrhea. Muscle twitching, weakness, tremor, incoordination, vomiting, abdominal cramps, and diarrhea all signal worsening of the poisoned state. Miosis is often a helpful diagnostic sign and the patient may report blurred and/or dark vision. Anxiety and restlessness are prominent, as are a few reports of choreaform movements. Psychiatric symptoms including depression, memory loss, and confusion have been reported. Toxic psychosis, manifested as confusion or bizarre behavior, has been misdiagnosed as alcohol intoxication.

Children will often present with a slightly different clinical picture than adults. Some of the typical cholinergic signs of bradycardia, muscular fasciculations, lacrimation, and sweating were less common. Seizures (22%–25%) and mental status changes including lethargy and coma (54%–96%) were common.[20, 21] In comparison, only 2-3% of adults present with seizures. Other common presenting signs in children include flaccid muscle weakness, miosis, and excessive salivation. In one study, 80% of cases were transferred with the wrong preliminary diagnosis.[20] In a second study, 88% of the parents initially denied any exposure history.[21]

See the preceding Toxicology section for information regarding the features of the intermediate syndrome and OPIDN.

Confirmation of Poisoning

If poisoning is probable, **treat the patient immediately. Do not wait for laboratory confirmation.**

Blood samples should be drawn to measure plasma pseudocholinesterase and red blood cell AChE levels. Depressions of plasma pseudocholinesterase and/or RBC acetylcholinersterase enzyme activities are generally available biochemical indicators of excessive organophosphate absorption. Certain organo-

---

APPROXIMATE LOWER LIMITS OF NORMAL PLASMA AND RED CELL CHOLINESTERASE ACTIVITIES IN HUMANS*

Methods	Plasma	RBC	Blood	Whole units
pH (Michel)	0.45	0.55		ΔpH per mL per hr
pH Stat (Nabb-Whitfield)	2.3	8.0		µM per mL per min
BMC Reagent Set (Ellman-Boehringer)	1,875		3,000	mU per mL per min
Dupont ACA	<8			Units per mL
Garry-Routh (Micro)			Male 7.8 Female 5.8	µM-SH per 3mL per min
Technicon	2.0	8.0		µM per mL per min

* Because measurement technique varies among laboratories, more accurate estimates of minimum normal values are usually provided by individual laboratories.

---

phosphates may selectively inhibit either plasma pseudocholinesterase or RBC acetylcholinesterase.[22] A minimum amount of organophosphate must be absorbed to depress blood cholinesterase activities, but enzyme activities, especially plasma pseudocholinesterase, may be lowered by dosages considerably less than are required to cause symptomatic poisoning. The enzyme depression is usually apparent within a few minutes or hours of significant absorption of organophosphate. Depression of the plasma enzyme generally persists several days to a few weeks. The RBC enzyme activity may not reach its minimum for several days, and usually remains depressed longer, sometimes 1–3 months, until new enzyme replaces that inactivated by organophosphate. The above table lists approximate lower limits of normal plasma and RBC cholinesterase activities of human blood, measured by several methods. **Lower levels usually indicate excessive absorption of a cholinesterase-inhibiting chemical.**

In certain conditions, the activities of plasma and RBC cholinesterase are depressed in the absence of chemical inhibition. About 3% of individuals have a genetically determined low level of plasma pseudocholinesterase. These persons are particularly vulnerable to the action of the muscle-paralyzing drug succinylcholine (often administered to surgical patients), but not to organophosphates. Patients with hepatitis, cirrhosis, malnutrition, chronic alcoholism, and dermatomyositis exhibit low plasma cholinesterase activities. A number of toxicants, notably cocaine, carbon disulfide, benzalkonium salts, organic mercury compounds, ciguatoxins, and solanines may reduce plasma pseudocholinesterase activity. Early pregnancy, birth control pills, and metoclopramide may also cause some depression. The RBC acetylcholinesterase is less likely than the plasma enzyme to be affected by factors other than organophosphates. It is, however, reduced in certain rare conditions that damage the red cell membrane, such as hemolytic anemia.

The alkyl phosphates and phenols to which organophosphates are hydrolyzed in the body can often be detected in the urine during pesticide absorption and up to about 48 hours thereafter. These analyses are sometimes useful in identifying and quantifying the actual pesticide to which workers have been exposed. Urinary alkyl phosphate and phenol analyses can demonstrate organophosphate absorption at lower dosages than those required to depress cholinesterase activities and at much lower dosages than those required to produce symptoms and signs. Their presence may simply be a result of organophosphates in the food chain.

Detection of intact organophosphates in the blood is usually not possible except during or soon after absorption of a substantial amount. In general, organophosphates do not remain unhydrolyzed in the blood for more than a few minutes or hours, unless the quantity absorbed is large or the hydrolyzing liver enzymes are inhibited.

Treatment

Caution: Persons attending the victim should avoid direct contact with heavily contaminated clothing and vomitus. Wear rubber gloves while washing pesticide from skin and hair. Vinyl gloves provide no protection.

1. Airway protection. Ensure that a clear airway exists. Intubate the patient and aspirate the secretions with a large-bore suction device if necessary. Administer oxygen by mechanically assisted pulmonary ventilation if respiration is depressed. **Improve tissue oxygenation as much as possible before administering atropine, so as to minimize the risk of ventricular fibrillation.** In severe poisonings, it may be necessary to support pulmonary ventilation mechanically for several days.

2. Atropine sulfate. Administer atropine sulfate intravenously, or intramuscularly if intravenous injection is not possible. Remember that atropine can be administered through an endotracheal tube if initial IV access is difficult to obtain. Depending on the severity of poisoning, doses of atropine ranging from very low to as high as 300 mg per day may be required,[23] or even continuous infusion.[24,25] (See dosage on next page.)

The objective of atropine antidotal therapy is to antagonize the effects of excessive concentrations of acetylcholine at end-organs having muscarinic receptors. Atropine does not reactivate the cholinesterase enzyme or accelerate disposition of organophosphate. Recrudescence of poisoning may occur if tissue concentrations of organophosphate remain high when the effect of atropine wears off. Atropine is effective against muscarinic manifestations, but it is ineffective against nicotinic actions, specifically muscle weakness and twitching, and respiratory depression.

Despite these limitations, atropine is often a life-saving agent in organophosphate poisonings. Favorable response to a test dose of atropine (1 mg in adults, 0.01 mg/kg in children under 12 years) can help differentiate poisoning by anticholinesterase agents from other conditions. However, lack of response, with no evidence of atropinization (atropine refractoriness) is typical of more severe poisonings. The adjunctive use of nebulized atropine has been reported to improve respiratory distress, decrease bronchial secretions, and increase oxygenation.[26]

3. Glycopyrolate has been studied as an alternative to atropine and found to have similar outcomes using continuous infusion. Ampules of 7.5 mg of glycopyrolate were added to 200 mL of saline and this infusion was titrated to the desired effects of dry mucous membranes and heart rate above 60 beats/min. During this study, atropine was used as a bolus for a heart rate less than 60 beats/min. The other apparent advantage to this regimen was a decreased number of respiratory infections. This may represent an alternative when there is a concern for respiratory infection due to excessive and difficult to control secretions, and in the presence of altered level of consciousness where the distinction between atropine toxicity or relapse of organophosphate poisoning is unclear.[27]

4. Pralidoxime. Before administration of pralidoxime, draw a blood sample (heparinized) for cholinesterase analysis (since pralidoxime tends to reverse the cholinesterase depression). Administer pralidoxime (Protopam, 2-PAM) a cholinesterase reactivator, in cases of severe poisoning by organophosphate pesticides in which respiratory depression, muscle weakness, and/or twitching are severe. (See dosage table on page 43.) When administered early (usually less than 48 hours after poisoning), pralidoxime relieves the nicotinic as well as the muscarinic effects of poisoning. Pralidoxime works by reactivating the cholinesterase and also by slowing the "aging" process of phosphorylated cholinesterase to a non-reactivatable form.

Note: Pralidoxime is of limited value and may actually be hazardous in poisonings by the cholinesterase-inhibiting carbamate compounds (see Chapter 5).

Dosage of Atropine:

In *moderately severe poisoning* (hypersecretion and other end-organ manifestations without central nervous system depression), the following dosage schedules have been used:

- *Adults and children over 12 years:* 2.0-4.0 mg, repeated every 15 minutes until pulmonary secretions are controlled, which may be accompanied by other signs of atropinization, including flushing, dry mouth, dilated pupils, and tachycardia (pulse of 140 per minute). **Warning:** In cases of ingestion of liquid concentrates of organophosphate pesticides, hydrocarbon aspiration may complicate these poisonings. Pulmonary edema and poor oxygenation in these cases will not respond to atropine and should be treated as a case of acute respiratory distress syndrome.

- *Children under 12 years:* 0.05-0.1 mg/kg body weight, repeated every 15 minutes until atropinization is achieved. There is a minimum dose of 0.1 mg in children. Maintain atropinization by repeated doses based on recurrence of symptoms for 2-12 hours or longer depending on severity of poisoning.

Maintain atropinization with repeated dosing as indicated by clinical status. Crackles in the lung bases nearly always indicate inadequate atropinization. Pulmonary improvement may not parallel other signs of atropinization. Continuation of, or return of, cholinergic signs indicates the need for more atropine. When symptoms are stable for as much as six hours, the dosing may be decreased.

Severely poisoned individuals may exhibit remarkable tolerance to atropine; two or more times the dosages suggested above may be needed. The dose of atropine may be increased and the dosing interval decreased as needed to control symptoms. Continuous intravenous infusion of atropine may be necessary when atropine requirements are massive. **The desired end-point is the reversal of muscarinic symptoms and signs with improvement in pulmonary status and oxygenation,** without an arbitrary dose limit. Preservative-free atropine products should be used whenever possible.

Note: Persons not poisoned or only slightly poisoned by organophosphates may develop signs of atropine toxicity from such large doses. Fever, muscle fibrillations, and delirium are the main signs of atropine toxicity. If these appear while the patient is fully atropinized, atropine administration should be discontinued, at least temporarily, while the severity of poisoning is reevaluated.

Dosage of pralidoxime may be repeated in 1-2 hours, then at 10-12 hour intervals if needed. In very severe poisonings, dosage rates may be doubled. Repeated doses of pralidoxime are usually required. In cases that involve continuing absorption of organophosphate (as after ingestion of large amount), or continuing transfer of highly lipophilic organophosphate from fat into blood, it may be necessary to continue administration of pralidoxime for several days beyond the 48 hour post-exposure interval usually cited as the limit of its effectiveness. Pralidoxime may also be given as a continuous infusion of approximately 500 mg/hour based on animal case studies and adult patient reports.[28,29]

Blood pressure should be monitored during administration because of the occasional occurrence of hypertensive crisis. Administration should be slowed or stopped if blood pressure rises to hazardous levels. Be prepared to assist pulmonary ventilation mechanically if respiration is depressed during or after pralidoxime administration. If intravenous injection is not possible, pralidoxime may be given by deep intramuscular injection.

5. Skin decontamination. In patients who have been poisoned by organophosphate contamination of skin, clothing, hair, and/or eyes, decontamination must proceed concurrently with whatever resuscitative and antidotal measures are necessary to preserve life. Flush the chemical from the eyes with copious amounts of clean water. If no symptoms are evident in a patient who remains alert and physically stable, a prompt shower and shampoo may be appropriate, provided the patient is carefully observed to insure against any sudden appearance of poisoning. If there are any indications of weakness, ataxia, or other neurologic impairment, clothing should be removed and a complete bath and shampoo given while the victim is recumbent, using copious amounts of soap and water. Attendants should wear rubber gloves as vinyl provides no protection against skin absorption. Surgical green soap is excellent for this purpose, but ordinary soap is about as good. Wash the chemical from skin folds and from under fingernails.

Contaminated clothing should be promptly removed, bagged, and laundered before returning. Contaminated leather shoes should be discarded. Note that the pesticide can contaminate the inside surfaces of gloves, boots, and headgear.

6. Gastrointestinal decontamination. If organophosphate has been ingested in quantity probably sufficient to cause poisoning, consideration should be given to gastrointestinal decontamination, as outlined in Chapter 2, General Principles. If the patient has already vomited, which is most likely in serious exposures, further efforts at GI decontamination may not be indicated. In significant ingestions, diarrhea and/or vomiting are so constant that charcoal adsorption and catharsis are not indicated.

7. Observation. Observe patient closely for at least 72 hours to ensure that symptoms (sweating, visual disturbances, vomiting, diarrhea, chest and abdominal distress, and sometimes pulmonary edema) do not recur as atropinization is withdrawn. In very severe poisonings by ingested organophosphates, particularly the more lipophilic and slowly hydrolyzed compounds, metabolic disposition of toxicant may require as many as 5-14 days. In some cases, this slow elimination may combine with profound cholinesterase inhibition to require atropinization for several days or even weeks. As dosage is reduced, the lung bases should be checked frequently for crackles. If crackles are heard, or if there is a return of miosis, bradycardia, sweating, or other cholinergic signs, atropinization must be re-established promptly.

8. Furosemide may be considered if pulmonary edema persists in the lungs even after full atropinization. It should not be used until the maximum benefit of atropine has been realized. Consult package insert for dosage and administration.

9. Pulmonary ventilation. Particularly in poisonings by large ingested doses of organophosphate, monitor pulmonary ventilation carefully, even after recovery from muscarinic symptomatology, to forestall respiratory failure. In some cases, respiratory failure has developed several days following organophosphate ingestion, and has persisted for days to weeks.

10. Hydrocarbon aspiration may complicate poisonings that involve ingestion of liquid concentrates of organophosphate pesticides. Pulmonary edema and poor oxygenation in these cases will not respond to atropine and should be treated as a case of acute respiratory distress syndrome.

11. Cardiopulmonary monitoring. In severely poisoned patients, monitor cardiac status by continuous ECG recording. Some organophosphates have significant cardiac toxicity.

12. Seizure control. Rarely, in severe organophosphate poisonings, convulsions occur despite therapy with atropine and pralidoxime. Insure that causes unrelated to pesticide toxicity are not responsible: head trauma, cerebral anoxia, or mixed poisoning. Drugs useful in controlling convulsions are discussed in Chapter 2. The benzodiazepines (diazepam or lorazepam) are the agents of choice as initial therapy.

13. Contraindications. The following drugs are contraindicated in nearly all organophosphate poisoning cases: morphine, succinylcholine, theophylline, phenothiazines, and reserpine. Adrenergic amines should be given only if there is a specific indication, such as marked hypotension.

14. Re-exposures. Persons who have been clinically poisoned by organophosphate pesticides should not be re-exposed to cholinesterase-inhibiting chemicals until symptoms and signs have resolved completely and blood cholinesterase activities have returned to at least 80 percent of pre-poisoning levels. If blood cholinesterase was not measured prior to poisoning, blood enzyme activities should reach at least minimum normal levels (see table on page 39) before the patient is returned to a pesticide-contaminated environment.

15. Do not administer atropine or pralidoxime prophylactically to workers exposed to organophosphate pesticides. Prophylactic dosage with either atropine or pralidoxime may mask early signs and symptoms of organophosphate poisoning and thus allow the worker to continue exposure and possibly progress to more severe poisoning. Atropine itself may enhance the health hazards of the agricultural work setting: impaired heat loss due to reduced sweating and impaired ability to operate mechanical equipment due to blurred vision. This can be caused by mydriasis, one of the effects of atropine.

General Chemical Structure

R is usually either ethyl or methyl. The insecticides with a double bonded sulfur are organothiophosphates, but are converted to organophosphates in the liver. Phosphonate contains an alkyl (R-) in place of one alkoxy group (RO-). "X" is called the "leaving group" and is the principal metabolite for a specific identification.

RO   S (or O)
   \ /
    P
   / \
RO   O
          Leaving Group

References

1. DuBois KP. The toxicity of organophosphorous compounds to mammals. *Bull World Health Organ* 1971;44:233-40.

2. Pasquet J, Mazuret A, Fournel J, et al. Acute oral and percutaneous toxicity of phosalone in the rat, in comparison with azinphosmethyl and parathion. *Toxicol Appl Pharmacol* 1976;37:85-92.

3. Garcia-Repetto R, Martinez D, and Repetto M. Coefficient of distribution of some organo-phosphorus pesticides in rat tissue. *Vet Hum Toxicol* 1995;37:226-9.

4. Gallo MA and Lawryk NJ. Organic phosphorus pesticides. In: Haves WJ and Laws ER (eds), Handbook of Pesticide Toxicology, vol 2, Classes of Pesticides. San Diego, CA: Academic Press Inc., 1991.

5. Taylor P. Anticholinesterase agents. In: Gilman AG and Goodman LS (eds), The Pharmaco-logical Basis of Therapeutics. New York: Macmillan Publishing Co. Inc.; 1985, pp.110-28.

6. De Kort WL, Kiestra SH, and Sangster B. The use of atropine and oximes in organophos-phate intoxications: A modified approach. *Clin Toxicol* 1988;26:199-208.

7. Jamal JA. Neurological syndromes of organophosphorus compounds. *Adverse Drug React Toxicol Rev* 1997;16(3):133-70.

8. Steenland K, Jenkins B, Ames RG, et al. Chronic neurological sequelae to organophosphate poisoning. *Am J Public Health* 1994;84:731-6.

9. Savage E, Keefe T, Mounce L, et al. Chronic neurological sequelae of acute organophosphate pesticide poisoning. *Arch Environ Health* 1988;43:38-45.

10. Rosenstock L, Keifer M, Daniell W, et al. Chronic central nervous system effects of acute organophosphate pesticide intoxication. *Lancet* 1991;338:223-7.

11. Gershon S and Shaw FH. Psychiatric sequelae of chronic exposure to organophosphorus insecticides. *Lancet* 1961; 1:1371-4.

12. Metcalf DR and Holmes JH. EEG, psychological, and neurological alterations in humans with organophosphorus exposure. *Ann NY Acad Sci* 1969;160:357-65.

13. Holmes JH and Gaon MD. Observations on acute and multiple exposure to anticholinest-erase agents. *Trans Am Clin Climatol Assoc* 1957; 68:86-103.

14. Hirshberg A and Lerman Y. Clinical problems in organophosphate insecticide poisoning: The use of a computerized information system. *Fundam Appl Toxicol* 1984; 4:S209-14.

15. Miller CS and Mitzel HC. Chemical sensitivity attributed to pesticide exposure versus re-modeling. *Arch Environ Health* 1995; 50:119-29.

16. DeBleeker J, Willems J, Van Den Neucker K, et al. Prolonged toxicity with intermediate syndrome after combined parathion and methyl parathion poisoning. *Clin Toxicol* 1992;30:333-45.

17. DeBleecker J, Van Den Neucker K, and Colardyn F. Intermediate syndrome in organo-phosphorous poisoning: A prospective study. *Crit Care Med* 1993;21:1706-11.

18. Aldridge WN and Nemery B. Toxicology of trialkylphosphorothioates with particular reference to lung toxicity. *Fundam Appl Toxicol* 1984; 4:S215-23.

19. Bardin PG, Van Eeden SF, Moolman JA, et al. Organophosphate and carbamate poisoning. *Arch Intern Med* 1994;154:1433-41.

20. Zwiener RJ and Ginsburg CM. Organophosphate and carbamate poisoning in infants and children. *Pediatrics* 1988;81:121-683.

21. Sofer S, Tal A, and Shahak E. Carbamate and organophosphate poisoning in early childhood. *Pediatr Emerg Care* 1989;5(4):222-5.

22. Sullivan JB and Blose J. Organophosphate and carbamate insecticides. In: Sullivan JB and Krieger GR (eds), Hazardous Materials Toxicology. Baltimore, MD: Williams and Wilkins, 1992, pp. 1015-26.

23. Goswamy R, Chaudhuri A, and Mahashur AA. Study of respiratory failure in organophosphate and carbamate poisoning. *Heart Lung* 1994;23:466-72.

24. LeBlanc FN, Benson BE, and Gilg AD. A severe organophosphate poisoning requiring the use of an atropine drip. *Clin Toxicol* 1986;24:69-76.

25. DuToit PW, Muller FO, Van Tonder WM, et al. Experience with the intensive care management of organophosphate insecticide poisoning. *S Afr Med J* 1981;60:227-9.

26. Shockley LW. The use of inhaled nebulized atropine for the treatment of malathion poisoning. *Clin Toxicol* 1989;27:183-92.

27. Bardin PG and van Eeden SF. Organophosphate poisoning: Grading the severity and comparing treatment between atropine and glycopyrrolate. *Crit Care Med* 1990;18:956-60.

28. Thompson DF, Thompson GD, Greenwood RB, et al. Therapeutic dosing of pralidoxime chloride. *Drug Intell Clin Pharm* 1987;21:590-2.

29. Tush GM and Anstead MI. Pralidoxime continuous infusion in the treatment of organophosphate poisoning. *Ann Pharmacother* 1997;31:441-4.

CHAPTER 5

N-Methyl Carbamate Insecticides

HIGHLIGHTS

- Cause reversible carbamylation of AChE
- Muscarinic, nicotinic, CNS effects

Signs and Symptoms:

- Malaise, muscle weakness, dizziness, sweating
- Headache, salivation, nausea, vomiting, abdominal pain, diarrhea
- CNS depression, pulmonary edema in serious cases

Treatment:

- Clear airway, improve tissue oxygenation
- Administer atropine sulfate intravenously
- Proceed immediately with decontamination procedures

N-Methyl carbamate insecticides are widely used in homes, gardens, and agriculture. They share with organophosphates the capacity to inhibit cholinesterase enzymes and therefore share similar symptomatology during acute and chronic exposures. Likewise, exposure can occur by several routes in the same individual due to multiple uses, and there is likely to be additive toxicity with simultaneous exposure to organophosphates. However, due to the somewhat different affinity for cholinesterases, as compared to organophosphates, these poisonings are often somewhat easier to treat, as discussed later in this chapter.

Toxicology

The N-methyl carbamate esters cause reversible carbamylation of the acetylcholinesterase enzyme, allowing accumulation of acetylcholine, the neuromediator substance, at parasympathetic neuroeffector junctions (muscarinic effects), at skeletal muscle myoneural junctions and autonomic ganglia (nicotinic effects), and in the brain (CNS effects). The carbamyl-acetylcholinesterase combination dissociates more readily than the phosphoryl-acetylcholinesterase complex produced by organophosphate compounds. This lability has several important consequences: (1) it tends to limit the duration of N-methyl carbamate poisonings, (2) it accounts for the greater span between symptom-producing and lethal doses than in most organophosphate compounds, and (3) it frequently invalidates the measurement of blood cholinesterase activity as a diagnostic index of poisoning (see below).

N-methyl carbamates are absorbed by inhalation and ingestion and somewhat by skin penetration, although the latter tends to be the less toxic route. For example, carbofuran has a rat oral LD_{50} of 5 mg/kg, compared to a rat dermal LD_{50} of 120 mg/kg, which makes the oral route approximately 24 times more toxic when ingested.[1] N-methyl carbamates are hydrolyzed enzymatically by the liver; degradation products are excreted by the kidneys and the liver.

At cholinergic nerve junctions with smooth muscle and gland cells, high acetylcholine concentration causes muscle contraction and secretion, respectively. At skeletal muscle junctions, excess acetylcholine may be excitatory (cause muscle twitching), but may also weaken or paralyze the cell by depolarizing the end-plate. In the brain, elevated acetylcholine concentrations may cause sensory and behavioral disturbances, incoordination, and depressed motor function (rarely seizures), even though the N-methyl carbamates do not penetrate the central nervous system very efficiently. Respiratory depression combined with pulmonary edema is the usual cause of death from poisoning by N-methyl carbamate compounds.

Signs and Symptoms of Poisoning

As with organophosphate poisoning, the signs and symptoms are based on excessive cholinergic stimulation. Unlike organophosphate poisoning, carbamate poisonings tend to be of shorter duration because the inhibition of nervous tissue AchE is reversible, and carbamates are more rapidly metabolized.[2] Bradycardia and seizures are less common than in organophosphate poisonings. However, **blood cholinesterase levels may be misleading due to in vitro reactivation of a carbamylated enzyme.**[3,4] A falsely "normal" level can make the diagnosis more difficult in the acute presentation in the absence of an exposure history.

The primary manifestations of serious toxicity are central nervous system depression, as manifested by coma, seizures, and hypotonicity, and nicotinic effects including hypertension and cardiorespiratory depression. Dyspnea, bronchospasm, and bronchorrhea with eventual pulmonary edema are other serious signs. Recent information indicates that children and adults differ in their clinical presentation. Children are more likely than adults to present with the CNS symptoms above. While children can still develop the classic muscarinic signs, the absence of them does not exclude the possibility of carbamate poisoning in the presence of CNS depression.[5]

Malaise, muscle weakness, dizziness, and sweating are commonly reported early symptoms. Headache, salivation, nausea, vomiting, abdominal pain, and diarrhea are often prominent. Miosis with blurred vision, incoordination, muscle twitching, and slurred speech are reported.

Confirmation of Poisoning

If there are strong clinical indications of acute N-methyl carbamate poisoning, and/or a history of carbamate exposure, treat the patient immediately. Do not wait for laboratory confirmation.

Blood for plasma pseudocholinesterase and RBC AChE should be obtained. Be advised that unless a substantial amount of N-methyl carbamate has been absorbed and a blood sample is taken within an hour or two, it is unlikely that blood cholinesterase activities will be found depressed. Even under the above circumstances, a rapid test for enzyme activity must be used to detect an effect, because enzyme reactivation occurs *in vitro* as well as *in vivo*. See the table on page 39 for methods of measurement of blood cholinesterase activities, if circumstances appear to warrant performance of the test.

aldicarb[+]
  Temik
aminocarb[+]
  Matacil
bendiocarb[+]
  Dycarb
  Ficam
  Multamat
  Niomil
  Tattoo
  Turcam
bufencarb
  Bux
  metalkamate
carbaryl
  Dicarbam
  Sevin
carbofuran[+]
  Crisfuran
  Curaterr
  Furadan
cloethocarb[+]
  Lance
dimetan
  Dimethan
dioxacarb
  Elecron
  Famid
fenoxycarb
  Torus
formetanate hydrochloride[+]
  Carzol
isolan[+]
  Primin
isoprocarb
  Etrofolan
  MIPC
methiocarb[+]
  Draza
  Mesurol
methomyl[+]
  Lannate
  Lanox
  Nudrin
mexacarbate
  Zectran
oxamyl[+]
  DPX 1410
  Vydate L
pirimicarb
  Abol
  Aficida
  Aphox
  Fernos
  Pirimor
  Rapid

(Continued on the next page)

promecarb
  Carbamult
propoxur
  aprocarb
  Baygon
thiodicarb
  Larvin
trimethacarb
  Broot
  Landrin

+ Indicates high toxicity. Highly toxic N-methyl carbamates have listed oral LD_{50} values (rat) less than or equal to 50 mg/kg body weight. Most other carbamates included in this table are considered moderately toxic, with LD_{50} values in excess of 50 mg/kg and less than 500 mg/kg.

Absorption of some N-methyl carbamates can be confirmed by analysis of urine for unique metabolites: alpha-naphthol from carbaryl, isopropoxyphenol from propoxur, carbofuran phenol from carbofuran, and aldicarb sulfone, sulfoxide, and nitrile from aldicarb. These complex analyses, when available, can be useful in identifying the responsible agent and following the course of carbamate disposition.

Treatment

Caution: Persons attending the victim should avoid direct contact with heavily contaminated clothing and vomitus. Wear rubber gloves while washing pesticide from skin and hair. Vinyl gloves provide no protection.

1. Airway protection. Ensure that a clear airway exists. Intubate the patient and aspirate the secretions with a large-bore suction device if necessary. Administer oxygen by mechanically assisted pulmonary ventilation if respiration is depressed. **Improve tissue oxygenation as much as possible before administering atropine, to minimize the risk of ventricular fibrillation.** In severe poisonings, it may be necessary to support pulmonary ventilation mechanically for several days.

2. Atropine. Administer atropine sulfate intravenously, or intramuscularly if intravenous injection is not possible. Remember that atropine can be administered through an endotracheal tube if initial IV access is difficult to obtain. Carbamates usually reverse with much smaller dosages of atropine than those required to reverse organophosphates.[6] (See dosage on next page.)

The objective of atropine antidotal therapy is to antagonize the effects of excessive concentrations of acetylcholine at end-organs having muscarinic receptors. Atropine does not reactivate the cholinesterase enzyme or accelerate excretion or breakdown of carbamate. Recrudescence of poisoning may occur if tissue concentrations of toxicant remain high when the effect of atropine wears off. Atropine is effective against muscarinic manifestations, but is ineffective against nicotinic actions, specifically, muscle weakness and twitching, and respiratory depression.

Despite these limitations, atropine is often a life-saving agent in N-methyl carbamate poisonings. Favorable response to a test dose of atropine (1 mg in adults, 0.01 mg/kg in children under 12 years) given intravenously can help differentiate poisoning by anticholinesterase agents from other conditions such as cardiogenic pulmonary edema and hydrocarbon ingestion. However, lack of response to the test dose, indicating no atropinization (atropine refractoriness), is characteristic of moderately severe to severe poisoning and indicates a need for further atropine. If the test dose does not result in mydriasis and drying of secretions, the patient can be considered atropine refractory.

Dosage of Atropine:

In *moderately severe poisoning* (hypersecretion and other end-organ manifestations without central nervous system depression), the following dosage schedules have proven effective:

- *Adults and children over 12 years:* 2.0-4.0 mg, repeated every 15 minutes until pulmonary secretions are controlled, which may be accompanied by other signs of atropinization, including flushing, dry mouth, dilated pupils, and tachycardia (pulse of 140 per minute). **Warning:** In cases of ingestion of liquid concentrates of carbamate pesticides, hydrocarbon aspiration may complicate these poisonings. Pulmonary edema and poor oxygenation in these cases will not respond to atropine and should be treated as a case of acute respiratory distress syndrome.

- *Children under 12 years:* 0.05-0.1 mg/kg body weight, repeated every 15 minutes until pulmonary secretions are controlled, which may be accompanied by other signs of atropinization as above (heart rates vary depending on age of child with young toddlers having a rate approaching 200). There is a minimum dose of 0.1 mg in children.

Maintain atropinization by repeated doses based on recurrence of symptoms for 2-12 hours or longer depending on severity of poisoning. Crackles in the lung bases nearly always indicate inadequate atropinization and pulmonary improvement may not parallel other signs. Continuation or return of cholinergic signs indicates the need for more atropine.

Severely poisoned individuals may exhibit remarkable tolerance to atropine; two or more times the dosages suggested above may be needed. Reversal of muscarinic manifestations, rather than a specific dosage, is the object of atropine therapy. However, prolonged intensive intravenous administration of atropine sometimes required in organophosphate poisonings is rarely needed in treating carbamate poisoning.

Note: Persons not poisoned or only slightly poisoned by N-methyl carbamates may develop signs of atropine toxicity from such large doses. Fever, muscle fibrillations, and delirium are the main signs of atropine toxicity. If these signs appear while the patient is fully atropinized, atropine administration should be discontinued, at least temporarily, while the severity of poisoning is reevaluated.

3. Skin decontamination. In patients with contaminated skin, clothing, hair, and/or eyes, **decontamination must proceed concurrently with whatever resuscitative and antidotal measures are needed to preserve life.** Flush the chemical from eyes with copious amounts of clean water. For asymptomatic individuals who are alert and physically able, a prompt shower and shampoo may be appropriate for thorough skin decontamination, provided the patient is carefully observed to insure against sudden appearance of poisoning. If there are any indications of weakness ataxia or other neurologic impairment, clothing should be removed and a complete bath and shampoo given while the victim is recumbent, using copious amounts of soap and water. Attendants should wear rubber gloves as vinyl provides no protection against skin absorption. Wash the chemical from skin folds and from under fingernails.

Contaminated clothing should be promptly removed, bagged, and laundered before returning. Contaminated leather shoes should be discarded. Note that the pesticide can contaminate the inside surfaces of gloves, boots, and headgear.

4. Gastrointestinal decontamination. If N-methyl carbamate has been ingested in a quantity probably sufficient to cause poisoning, consideration should be given to gastrointestinal decontamination as outlined in Chapter 2. If the patient has presented with a recent ingestion and is still asymptomatic, adsorption of poison with activated charcoal may be beneficial. In significant ingestions, diarrhea and/or vomiting are so constant that charcoal adsorption and catharsis are not indicated. Attention should be given to oxygen, airway management, and atropine.

5. Urine sample. Save a urine sample for metabolite analysis if there is need to identify the agent responsible for the poisoning.

6. Pralidoxime is probably of little value in N-methyl carbamate poisonings, because atropine alone is effective. Although not indicated in isolated carbamate poisoning, pralidoxime appears to be useful in cases of mixed carbamate/organophosphate poisonings, and cases of an unknown pesticide with muscarinic symptoms on presentation.[7,8] See Chapter 4, Treatment section, p. 41.

7. Observation. Observe patient closely for at least 24 hours to ensure that symptoms (sweating, visual disturbances, vomiting, diarrhea, chest and abdominal distress, and sometimes pulmonary edema) do not recur as atropinization is withdrawn. The observation period should be longer in the case of a mixed pesticide ingestion, because of the prolonged and delayed symptoms associated with organophosphate poisoning. As the dosage of atropine is reduced over time, check the lung bases frequently for crackles. Atropinization must be re-established promptly, if crackles are heard, or if there is a return of miosis, sweating, or other signs of poisoning.

8. Furosemide may be considered for relief of pulmonary edema if crackles persist in the lungs even after full atropinization. It should not be considered until the maximum effect of atropine has been achieved. Consult package insert for dosage and administration.

9. Pulmonary ventilation. Particularly in poisonings by large doses of N-methyl carbamates, monitor pulmonary ventilation carefully, even after recovery from muscarinic symptomatology, to forestall respiratory failure.

10. Cardiopulmonary monitoring. In severely poisoned patients, monitor cardiac status by continuous ECG recording.

11. Contraindications. The following drugs are probably contraindicated in nearly all N-methyl carbamate poisoning cases: morphine, succinlycholine, theophylline, phenothiazines, and reserpine. Adrenergic amines should be given only if there is a specific indication, such as marked hypotension.

12. Hydrocarbon aspiration may complicate poisonings that involve ingestion of liquid concentrates of some carbamates that are formulated in a petroleum product base. Pulmonary edema and poor oxygenation in these cases will not respond to atropine and should be treated as cases of acute respiratory distress syndrome.

13. Do not administer atropine prophylactically to workers exposed to N-methyl carbamate pesticides. Prophylactic dosage may mask early symptoms and signs of carbamate poisoning and thus allow the worker to continue exposure and possibly progress to more severe poisoning. Atropine itself may enhance the health hazards of the agricultural work setting: impaired heat loss due to reduced sweating and impaired ability to operate mechanical equipment due to blurred vision (mydriasis).

General Chemical Structure

$$H_3C \diagdown \underset{H}{\overset{}{N}} - \overset{\overset{O}{\|}}{C} - O - \boxed{\text{Leaving Group}}$$

References

1. Registry of Toxic Effects of Chemical Substances. National Institute for Occupational Safety and Health, Cincinnati, OH. (CD-ROM Version, Micromedex, Inc. Englewood, CA 1991.)

2. Ecobichon DJ. Toxic effect of pesticides. In: Klaassen CD (ed), Casarett & Doull's Toxicology: The Basic Science of Poisons, 5th ed. New York: McGraw-Hill, 1996, p. 659.

3. Rotenberg M and Almog S. Evaluation of the decarbamylation process of cholinesterase during assay of enzyme activity. *Clin Chim Acta* 1995;240:107-16.

4. Jokanovic M and Maksimovic M. Abnormal cholinesterase activity: Understanding and interpretation. *Eur J Clin Chem Clin Biochem* 1997;35:11-6.

5. Lifshitz M, Shahak E, Bolotin A, et al. Carbamate poisoning in early childhood and in adults. *Clin Toxicol* 1997;35:25-7.

6. Goswamy R et al. Study of respiratory failure in organophosphate and carbamate poisoning. *Heart Lung* 1994;23:466-72.

7. Lifshitz M, Totenberg M, Sofer S, et al. Carbamate poisoning and oxime treatment in children: A clinical and laboratory study. *Pediatrics* 1994;93:652-5.

8. Kurtz PH. Pralidoxime in the treatment of carbamate intoxication. *Am J Emerg Med* 1990;8:68-70.

Solid Organochlorine Insecticides

EPA has sharply curtailed the availability of many organochlorines, particularly DDT, aldrin, dieldrin, heptachlor, mirex, chlordecone, and chlordane. Others, however, remain the active ingredients of various home and garden products and some agricultural, structural, and environmental pest control products. Hexachlorobenzene is a fungicide used as a seed protectant and is discussed further in Chapter 15, Fungicides.

Technical hexachlorocyclohexane (misnamed benzene hexachloride, BHC) includes multiple stereoisomers; only the gamma isomer (lindane) is insecticidal. Lindane is the active ingredient of some pest control products used in the home and garden, on the farm, and in forestry and animal husbandry. It is also the active agent in the medicine Kwell®, used for human ectoparasitic disease. Lindane has been reported on numerous occasions to be associated with acute neurological toxicity either from ingestion or in persons treated for scabies or lice.[1-6]

Toxicology

In varying degrees, organochlorines are absorbed from the gut and also by the lung and across the skin. The efficiency of dermal absorption is variable. Hexachlorocyclohexane, including lindane, the cyclodienes (aldrin, dieldrin, endrin, chlordane, heptachlor), and endosulfan are efficiently absorbed across the skin, while dermal absorption efficiencies of DDT, dicofol, marlate, toxaphene, and mirex are substantially less.[7] Lindane has a documented 9.3% dermal absorption rate,[8] and is absorbed even more efficiently across abraded skin.[1,9] This becomes especially important when taking into account its use on children with severe dermatitis associated with scabies. Fat and fat solvents enhance gastrointestinal, and probably dermal, absorption of organochlorines. While most of the solid organochlorines are not highly volatile, pesticide-laden aerosol or dust particles trapped in respiratory mucous and subsequently swallowed may lead to significant gastrointestinal absorption.

Following exposure to some organochlorines (notably DDT), a significant part of the absorbed dose is stored in fat tissue as the unchanged parent compound. Most organochlorines are in some degree dechlorinated, oxidized, then conjugated. The chief route of excretion is biliary, although nearly all organochlorines yield measurable urinary metabolites. Unfortunately, many of the unmetabolized pesticides are efficiently reabsorbed by the intestine (enterohepatic circulation), substantially retarding fecal excretion.

Commercial Products

aldrin*
benzene hexachloride (BHC)*
  HCH
  hexachlor
  hexachloran
chlordane*
  (multiple trade names)
chlordecone*
  Kepone
chlorobenzilate
DDT*
  (multiple trade names)
dicofol
  Kelthane
  (multiple trade names)
dieldrin*
  Dieldrite
dienochlor
  Pentac
endosulfan
  (multiple trade names)
endrin*
  Hexadrin
heptachlor**
  (multiple trade names)
hexacholorobenzene*
lindane
  gamma BHC or HCH
  Kwell
  (multiple trade names)
methoxychlor
  Marlate
mirex*
terpene polychlorinates*
  Strobane
toxaphene*

  * All U.S. registrations have
     been cancelled.

  ** Registered in the United
     States only for
     underground use in
     power lines for fire ants.

Metabolic dispositions of DDT and DDE (a DDT degradation product), the beta isomer of hexachlorocyclohexane, dieldrin, heptachlor epoxide, and mirex tend to be slow, leading to storage in body fat. Storable lipophilic compounds are likely to be excreted in maternal milk.[6,10,11] On the other hand, rapid metabolic dispositions of lindane, methoxychlor, dienochlor, endrin, chlorobenzilate, dicofol, toxaphene, perthane, and endosulfan reduce the likelihood that these organochlorines will be detected as residues in body fat, blood, or milk.

The chief acute toxic action of organochlorine pesticides is on the nervous system, where these compounds induce a hyperexcitable state in the brain.[12] This effect is manifest mainly as convulsions, sometimes limited to myoclonic jerking, but often expressed as violent seizures. Convulsions caused by cyclodienes may recur over periods of several days. Other less severe signs of neurologic toxicity such as paresthesias, tremor, ataxia, and hyperreflexia are also characteristic of acute organochlorine poisoning. Agents such as DDT and methoxychlor tend to cause the less severe effects, while the cyclodienes, mirex, and lindane are associated with the more severe seizures and fatalities.[7] Convulsions may cause death by interfering with pulmonary gas exchange and by generating severe metabolic acidosis.

High tissue concentrations of organochlorines increase myocardial irritability, predisposing to cardiac arrhythmia. When tissue organochlorine concentrations drop below threshold levels, recovery from the poisoning occurs. Organochlorines are not cholinesterase inhibitors.

High tissue levels of some organochlorines (notably DDT, DDE, and cyclodienes) have been shown to induce hepatic microsomal drug-metabolizing enzymes.[13] This tends to accelerate excretion of the pesticides themselves, but may also stimulate biotransformation of critical natural substances, such as steroid hormones and therapeutic drugs, occasionally necessitating re-evaluation of required dosages in persons intensively exposed to organochlorines. Human absorption of organochlorine sufficient to cause enzyme induction is likely to occur only as a result of prolonged intensive exposure.

Ingestion of hexachlorobenzene-treated wheat has been associated with human dermal toxicity diagnosed as porphyria cutanea tarda. The skin blisters, becomes very sensitive to sunlight, and heals poorly, resulting in scarring and contracture formation.[14] Unlike other organochlorine compounds, there have been no reported cases of convulsions caused by the fungicide hexachlorobenzene. Lindane and chlordane have rarely been associated anecdotally with certain hematological disorders, including aplastic anemia and megaloblastic anemia.[15,16]

There has been considerable interest recently in the interaction of organochlorines with endocrine receptors, particularly estrogen and androgen receptors. *In vitro* studies and animal experimentation have supported the view that the function of the endocrine system may be altered by these interactions.[17,18] This in turn may alter the reproductive development and success of animals and humans. In addition, some organochlorines may inhibit lactation and may also be developmental toxicants.[10] Due to evidence of carcinogenic potential, some organochlorines have lost registration for use in the United States or had their uses restricted. Although these effects are important, they are beyond the scope of this manual.

Signs and Symptoms of Poisoning

Early manifestations of poisoning by some organochlorine pesticides, particularly DDT, are often sensory disturbances: hyperesthesia and paresthesia of the face and extremities. Headache, dizziness, nausea, vomiting, incoordination, tremor, and mental confusion are also reported. More severe poisoning causes myoclonic jerking movements, then generalized tonic-clonic convulsions. Coma and respiratory depression may follow the seizures.

Poisoning by the cyclodienes and toxaphene is more likely to begin with the sudden onset of convulsions, and is often not preceded by the premonitory manifestations mentioned above. Seizures caused by cyclodienes may appear as long as 48 hours after exposure, and then may recur periodically over several days following the initial episode. Because lindane and toxaphene are more rapidly biotransformed in the body and excreted, they are less likely than dieldrin, aldrin, and chlordane to cause delayed or recurrent seizures.

Confirmation of Poisoning

Organochlorine pesticides and/or their metabolites can sometimes be identified in blood by gas-liquid chromatographic examination of samples taken within a few days of significant pesticide absorption. Such tests are performed by a limited number of government, university, and private laboratories, which can usually be contacted through poison control centers or health departments. Some organochlorine pesticides or their products (notably DDT, dieldrin, mirex, heptachlor, epoxide, chlordecone) persist in tissues and blood for weeks or months after absorption, but others are likely to be excreted in a few days, limiting the likelihood of detection. Blood levels tend to correlate more with acute toxicity, while levels found in adipose tissue and breast milk usually reflect more long-term and historic exposure.[19]

Chromatographic methods make possible detection of most organochlorines at concentrations much lower than those associated with symptoms of toxicity. Therefore, a positive finding in a blood sample does not, of itself, justify a diagnosis of acute poisoning. Lindane appears in the literature more frequently than other compounds. The time of acquisition of the blood level in relation to exposure time must be taken into account when interpreting blood levels. In one study, lindane levels were measured at 10.3 ng/mL in healthy volunteers three days after application to the skin.[20]

In a study with childhood dermal absorption using children with scabies and a non-affected control group, lindane peaked at 28 ng/mL 6 hours after application in the affected group, and at 24 ng/mL in the control group. At 48 hours, levels were 6 ng/mL and 5 ng/mL respectively. Findings from this study also provide evidence for increased absorption across abraded skin.[9] A child with severely abraded skin was treated for scabies and developed seizures. Three days after exposure, his lindane level was 54 ng/mL.[1] Most reports of acute toxicity from lindane involve blood levels of 130 ng/mL or greater, with the most severe and fatal cases involving levels exceeding 500 ng/mL.[2]

DDT, DDE, and a few other organochlorines are still found at very low levels in blood samples from the general U.S. population, presumably due to past and/or current low-level contamination of food by these environmentally persistent pesticides.

In the absence of corresponding elevations of blood levels, the amount of stored pesticides is not likely to be of clinical significance. Measurements of urinary metabolites of some organochlorine pesticides can be useful in monitoring occupational exposures; however, the analytical methods are complex, and are not likely to detect amounts of metabolites generated by minimal exposures.

Treatment

1. Observation. Persons exposed to high levels of organochlorine pesticides by any route should be observed for sensory disturbances, incoordination, speech slurring, mental aberrations, and involuntary motor activity that would warn of imminent convulsions.

2. Convulsions. If convulsions occur, place the victim in the left lateral decubitus position with the head down. Move away furniture or other solid objects that could be a source of injury. If jaw movements are violent, place padded tongue blades between the teeth to protect the tongue. Whenever possible, remove dentures and other removable dental work. Aspirate oral and pharyngeal secretion, and when possible, insert an oropharyngeal airway to maintain an open passage unobstructed by the tongue. Minimize noise and any manipulation of the patient that may trigger seizure activity.

Dosage of Diazepam:

- *Adults*: 5–10 mg IV and repeat every 5–10 minutes to maximum of 30 mg.
- *Children*: 0.2 to 0.5 mg/kg every 5 minutes to maximum of 10 mg in children over 5 years, and maximum of 5 mg in children under 5 years.

Although lorazepam is widely accepted as a treatment of choice for status epilepticus, there are no reports of its use for organochlorine intoxication. Some cases have required aggressive seizure management including the addition of phenobarbital and the induction of pentobarbital coma.

Seizures in patients caused by organochlorine toxicity are likely to be prolonged and difficult to control. Status epilepticus is common. For this reason, patients with seizures that do not respond immediately to anticonvulsants should be transferred as soon as possible to a trauma center and will generally require intensive care admission until seizures are controlled and neurologic status is improved. Initial therapy with benzodiazepines should be instituted.

3. Oxygen. Administer oxygen by mask. Maintain pulmonary gas exchange by mechanically assisted ventilation whenever respiration is depressed.

4. Skin decontamination. Skin decontamination should be done thoroughly, as outlined in Chapter 2.

5. Gastrointestinal decontamination. If organochlorine has been ingested in a quantity sufficient to cause poisoning and the patient presents within an hour, consideration should be given to gastric decontamination procedures, as outlined in Chapter 2. If the patient presents more than an hour after ingestion, activated charcoal may still be beneficial. If the victim is convulsing, it is almost always necessary first to control seizures before attempting gastric decontamination. Activated charcoal administration has been advocated in such poisonings, but there is little human or experimental evidence to support it.

6. Respiratory failure. Particularly in poisonings by large doses of organochlorine, **monitor pulmonary ventilation** carefully to forestall respiratory failure. Assist pulmonary ventilation mechanically with oxygen whenever respiration is depressed. Since these compounds are often formulated in a hydrocarbon vehicle, hydrocarbon aspiration may occur with ingestion of these agents. The hydrocarbon aspiration should be managed in accordance with accepted medical practice as a case of acute respiratory distress syndrome which will usually require intensive care management.

7. Cardiac monitoring. In severely poisoned patients, monitor cardiac status by continuous ECG recording to detect arrhythmia.

8. Contraindications. Do not give epinephrine, other adrenergic amines, or atropine unless absolutely necessary because of the enhanced myocardial irritability induced by chlorinated hydrocarbons, which predisposes to ventricular fibrillation. Do not give animal or vegetable oils or fats by mouth. They enhance gastrointestinal absorption of the lipophilic organochlorines.

9. Phenobarbital. To control seizures and myoclonic movements that sometimes persist for several days following acute poisoning by the more slowly excreted organochlorines, phenobarbital given orally is likely to be effective.

Dosage should be based on manifestations in the individual case and on information contained in the package insert.

10. Cholestryamine resin accelerates the biliary-fecal excretion of the more slowly eliminated organochlorine compounds.[21] It is usually administered in 4 g doses, 4 times a day, before meals and at bedtime. The usual dose for children is 240 mg/kg/24 hours, divided Q 8 hours. The dose may be mixed with a pulpy fruit or liquid. It should never be given in its dry form and must always be administered with water, other liquids or a pulpy fruit. Prolonged treatment (several weeks or months) may be necessary.

11. Convalescence. During convalescence, enhance carbohydrate, protein, and vitamin intake by diet or parenteral therapy.

General Chemical Structures

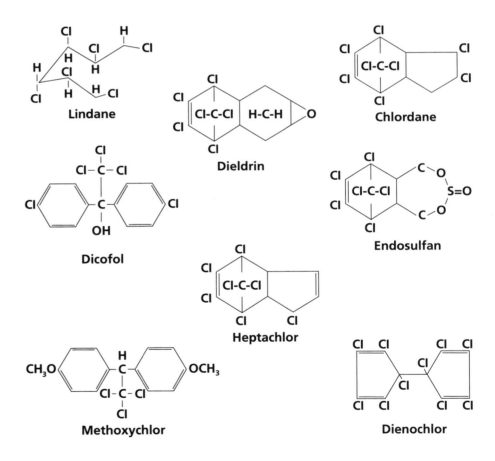

Lindane

Dieldrin

Chlordane

Dicofol

Endosulfan

Heptachlor

Methoxychlor

Dienochlor

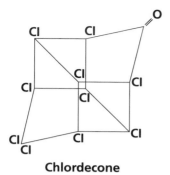

Chlordecone

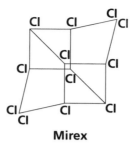

Mirex

References

1. Friedman SJ. Lindane neurotoxic reaction in nonbullous congenital ichthyosiform erythroderma. *Arch Dermatol* 1987;123:1056-8.

2. Aks SE, Krantz A, Hryhorczuk DO, et al. Acute accidental lindane ingestion in toddlers. *Ann Emerg Med* 1995;25(5):647-51.

3. Tenenbein M. Seizures after lindane therapy. *J Am Geriatr Soc* 1991;39(4):394-5.

4. Solomon BA, Haut SR, Carr EM, and Shalita AR. Neurotoxic reaction to lindane in an HIV-seropositive patient: An old medication's new problem. *J Fam Pract* 1995;40(3):291-6.

5. Fischer TF. Lindane toxicity in a 24-year-old woman. *Ann Emerg Med* 1994;24(5):972-4.

6. Solomon LM, Fahrner L, and West DP. Gamma benzene hexachloride toxicity. *Arch Dermatol* 1977;113:353-7.

7. Echobichon DJ. Toxic effects of pesticides. In Klaassen CD (ed), Casarett & Doull's Toxicology: The Basic Science of Poisons, 5th ed. New York: McGraw-Hill, 1996, pp. 649-55.

8. Feldmann RJ and Maibach HI. Percutaneous penetration of some pesticides and herbicides in man. *Toxicol and Appl Pharmacol* 1974;28:126-32.

9. Ginsburg CM, Lowry W, and Reisch JS. Absorption of lindane (gamma benzene hexachloride) in infants and children. *J Pediatr* 1997;91(6):998-1000.

10. Rogan WJ. Pollutants in breast milk. *Arch Pediatr Adolesc Med* 1996;150:981-90.

11. Stevens MF, Ebell GF, and Psaila-Savona P. Organochlorine pesticides in Western Australian nursing mothers. *Med J Aust* 1993;158(4):238-41.

12. Joy RM. The effects of neurotoxicants on kindling and kindled seizures. *Fundam Appl Toxicol* 1985;5:41-65.

13. Hunter J, Maxwell JD, Stewart DA, et al. Increased hepatic microsomal enzyme activity from occupational exposure to certain organochlorine pesticides. *Nature* 1972;237:399-401.

14. Booth NH and McDowell JR. Toxicity of hexachlorobenzene and associated residues in edible animal tissues. *J Am Vet Med Assoc* 1975;166(6):591-5.

15. Rauch AE, Kowalsky SF, Lesar TS, et al. Lindane (Kwell)-induced aplastic anemia. *Arch Intern Med* 1990;150:2393-5.

16. Furie B and Trubowitz S. Insecticides and blood dyscrasias. Chlordane exposure and self-limited refractory megaloblastic anemia. *JAMA* 1976;235(16):1720-2.

17. Vonier PM, Crain DA, McLachlan JA, et al. Interaction of environmental chemicals with the estrogen and progesterone receptors from the oviduct of the American alligator. *Environ Health Perspect* 1996;104(12):1318-22.

18. Fry DM. Reproductive effects in birds exposed to pesticides and industrial chemicals. *Environ Health Perspect* 1995;103(Suppl 7):165-71.

19. Frank R, Rasper J, Smout MS, and Braun HE. Organochlorine residues in adipose tissues, blood and milk from Ontario residents, 1976-1985. *Can J Public Health* 1988;79:150-8.

20. Hosler J, Tschan C, Hignite CE, et al. Topical application of lindane cream (Kwell) and antipyrine metabolism. *J Invest Dermatol* 1980;74:51-3.

21. Cohn WJ, Boylan JJ, Blanke RV, et al. Treatment of chlordecone (Kepone) toxicity with cholestyramine. *New Engl J Med* 1978;298(5):243-8.

CHAPTER 7

Biologicals and Insecticides of Biological Origin

This chapter covers several widely-used insecticidal products of natural origin, as well as certain agents often identified as biological control agents. Of the many living control agents, only the bacterial agent *Bacillus thuringiensis* will be discussed in detail, since it is one of the most widely used. Many other agents, such as parasitic wasps and insects, are so host-specific that they pose little or no risk to human health. The agents are discussed in this chapter in alphabetic order.

AZADIRACHTIN

This biologically-obtained insecticide is derived from the Neem tree (*Azadirachta indica*). It is an insect growth regulator that interferes with the molting hormone ecdysone.

Toxicology

Azadirachtin causes severe dermal and gastrointestinal irritation. Central nervous system stimulation and depression have been seen. This agent is primarily used and manufactured in India; little use or exposures are expected in the United States.

Treatment

1. Skin decontamination. If skin exposure occurs, the skin should be thoroughly washed with soap and water.

2. Gastrointestinal decontamination. Due to the severe gastrointestinal irritation, gastric emptying and catharsis are not indicated. Consideration should be given to administration of activated charcoal as outlined in Chapter 2.

HIGHLIGHTS

- Derived from living systems
- *Bacillus thuringensis* is the most important live agent
- Generally of low order toxicity

Signs and Symptoms:

- Highly variable based on specific agents
- Several cause gastrointestinal irritation
- Nicotine and rotenone may have serious CNS effects
- Nicotine and sabadilla may have cardiovascular effects

Treatment:

- Specific to the agent
- Skin, eye, and GI decontamination may be indicated
- Nicotine, rotenone, and sabadilla require aggressive support

(Continued on the next page)

BACILLUS THURINGIENSIS

Several strains of *Bacillus thuringiensis* are pathogenic to some insects. The bacterial organisms are cultured, then harvested in spore form for use as insecticide. Production methods vary widely. Proteinaceous and nucleotide-like toxins generated by the vegetative forms (which infect insects) are responsible for the insecticidal effect. The spores are formulated as wettable powders, flowable concentrates, and granules for application to field crops and for control of mosquitoes and black flies.

Toxicology

The varieties of *Bacillus thuringiensis* used commercially survive when injected into mice, and at least one of the purified insecticidal toxins is toxic to mice. Infections of humans have been extremely rare. A single case report of ingestion by volunteers of *Bacillus thuringiensis var. galleriae* resulted in fever and gastrointestinal symptoms. However, this agent is not registered as a pesticide. *B. thuringiensis* products are exempt from tolerance on raw agricultural commodities in the United States. Neither irritative nor sensitizing effects have been reported in workers preparing and applying commercial products.

Treatment

1. Skin decontamination. Skin contamination should be removed with soap and water. Eye contamination should be flushed from the eyes with clean water or saline. If irritation persists, or if there is any indication of infection, treatment by a physician should be obtained.

A single case of corneal ulcer caused by a splash of *B. thuringiensis* suspension into the eye was successfully treated by subconjunctival injection of gentamicin (20 mg) and cefazolin (25 mg).[1]

2. Gastrointestinal decontamination. If a *B. thuringiensis* product has been ingested, the patient should be observed for manifestations of bacterial gastroenteritis: abdominal cramps, vomiting, and diarrhea. The illness is likely to be self-limited if it occurs at all. The patient should be treated symptomatically and fluid support provided as appropriate.

EUGENOL

This compound is derived from clove oil. It is used as an insect attractant.

Toxicology

Eugenol is similar in its clinical effects to phenol. Although it works as an anesthetic, in large doses it can cause burns to epithelial surfaces.[2] Sloughing of mucous membranes has occurred as an allergic reaction to a small dose applied topically in the mouth.[3] Gastric mucosal lesions have been reported in animals, but no lesions were seen on endoscopy after clove oil ingestion.[4] Large doses may result in coma and liver dysfunction.[5]

Treatment

Treatment is primarily supportive as there is no antidote. If mucosal burns are present, consider endoscopy to look for other ulcerations.

GIBBERELLIC ACID (Gibberellin, GA_3)

Gibberellic acid is not a pesticide, but it is commonly used in agricultural production as a growth-promoting agent. It is a metabolic product of a cultured fungus, formulated in tablets, granules, and liquid concentrates for application to soil beneath growing plants and trees.

Toxicology

Experimental animals tolerate large oral doses without apparent adverse effect. No human poisonings have been reported. Sensitization has not been reported, and irritant effects are not remarkable.

Treatment

1. Skin decontamination. Wash contamination from skin with soap and water. Flush contamination from eyes with clean water or saline. If irritation occurs, obtain medical treatment.

2. Gastrointestinal decontamination. If gibberellic acid has been swallowed, there is no reason to expect adverse effects.

NICOTINE

Nicotine is an alkaloid contained in the leaves of many species of plants, but is usually obtained commercially from tobacco. A 14% preparation of the free alkaloid is marketed as a greenhouse fumigant. Significant volatilization of nicotine occurs. Commercial nicotine insecticides have long been known as Black Leaf 40. This formulation was discontinued in 1992. Other currently available formulations include dusts formulated with naphthalene and dried blood used to repel dogs and rabbits. Be aware of Green Tobacco Syndrome from dermal absorption. Very little nicotine insecticide is currently used in the United States, although old preparations of nicotine insecticides may still be found on occasion.[6] Today, most nicotine poisonings are the result of ingestion of tobacco products and incorrect use of nicotine skin patches.

Toxicology

Nicotine alkaloid is efficiently absorbed by the gut, lung, and skin. Extensive biotransformation occurs in the liver with 70–75% occurring as a first pass effect.[7] Both the liver and kidney participate in the formation and excretion of multiple end-products, which are excreted within a few hours. Estimates of the half-life of nicotine range from about one hour in smokers to as much as two hours in non-smokers.[8,9]

Toxic action is complex. At low doses, autonomic ganglia are stimulated. Higher doses result in blockade of autonomic ganglia and skeletal muscle neuromuscular junctions, and direct effects on the central nervous system. Paralysis and vascular collapse are prominent features of acute poisoning, but death is often due to respiratory paralysis, which may ensue promptly after the first symptoms of poisoning. Nicotine is not an inhibitor of the cholinesterase enzyme.

Signs and Symptoms of Poisoning

Early and prominent symptoms of poisoning include salivation, sweating, dizziness, nausea, vomiting, and diarrhea. Burning sensations in the mouth and throat, agitation, confusion, headache, and abdominal pain are reported. If dosage has been high, vascular collapse with hypotension, bradycardia or other arrythmias, dyspnea then respiratory failure, and unconsciousness may ensue promptly.[6,10,11,12] In some cases, hypertension and tachycardia may precede hypotension and bradycardia, with the latter two signs leading to shock.[11,12] Seizures may also occur.[6,11] In one case of ingestion of a large dose of nicotine alkaloid pesticide, the patient developed asystole within two minutes. He later developed seizures and refractory hypotension.[6]

Confirmation of Poisoning

Urine content of the metabolite cotinine can be used to confirm absorption of nicotine.

Treatment

1. Skin decontamination. If liquid or aerosol spray has come in contact with skin, wash the area thoroughly with soap and water. If eyes have been contaminated, flush them thoroughly with clean water or saline. If irritation persists, obtain specialized medical treatment.

If symptoms of poisoning appear during exposure to an airborne nicotine insecticide, remove the person from the contaminated environment immediately, wash any skin areas that may be contaminated, then transport the victim to the nearest treatment facility. Although mild poisoning may resolve without treatment, it is often difficult to predict the ultimate severity of poisoning at the onset.

2. Pulmonary ventilation. If there is any indication of loss of respiratory drive, maintain pulmonary ventilation by mechanical means, using supplemental oxygen if available, or mouth-to-mouth or mouth-to-nose methods if necessary. Toxic effects of nicotine other than respiratory depression are usually survivable. The importance of maintaining adequate gas exchange is therefore paramount.

3. Gastrointestinal decontamination. If a nicotine-containing product has been ingested recently, immediate steps must be taken to limit gastrointestinal absorption. If the patient is fully alert, immediate oral administration of activated charcoal as outlined in Chapter 2 is probably the best initial step in management. Repeated administration of activated charcoal at half or more the initial dosage every 2-4 hours may be beneficial. Since diarrhea is often a part of this poisoning, it is usually not necessary or appropriate to administer a cathartic. Do not administer syrup of ipecac.

4. Cardiac monitoring. Monitor cardiac status by electrocardiography, and measure blood pressure frequently. **Cardiopulmonary resuscitation may be necessary.** Vascular collapse may require administration of norepinephrine and/or dopamine. Consult package inserts for dosages and routes of administration. Infusions of electrolyte solutions, plasma, and/or blood may also be required to combat shock.

5. Atropine sulfate. There is no specific antidote for nicotine poisoning. Severe hypersecretion (especially salivation and diarrhea) or bradycardia may be treated with intravenous atropine sulfate. See dosage on next page.

> **Dosage of Atropine Sulfate:**
>
> - *Adults and children over 12 years:* 0.4-0.5 mg slowly IV, repeated every 5 minutes if necessary.
>
> - *Children under 12 years:* 0.01 mg/kg body weight, slowly IV, repeated every 5 minutes if necessary. There is a minimum dose of 0.1 mg.

6. Convulsions should be controlled as outlined in Chapter 2. If the patient survives for four hours, complete recovery is likely.

PYRETHRUM AND PYRETHRINS

Pyrethrum is the oleoresin extract of dried chrysanthemum flowers. The extract contains about 50% active insecticidal ingredients known as pyrethrins. The ketoalcoholic esters of chrysanthemic and pyrethroic acids are known as pyrethrins, cinerins, and jasmolins. These strongly lipophilic esters rapidly penetrate many insects and paralyze their nervous systems. Both crude pyrethrum extract and purified pyrethrins are contained in various commercial products, commonly dissolved in petroleum distillates. Some are packaged in pressurized containers ("bug-bombs"), usually in combination with the synergists piperonyl butoxide and n-octyl bicycloheptene dicarboximide. The synergists retard enzymatic degradation of pyrethrins. Some commercial products also contain organophosphate or carbamate insecticides. These are included because the rapid paralytic effect of pyrethrins on insects ("quick knockdown") is not always lethal.

Pyrethrum and pyrethrin products are used mainly for indoor pest control. They are not sufficiently stable in light and heat to remain as active residues on crops. The synthetic insecticides known as pyrethroids (chemically similar to pyrethrins) do have the stability needed for agricultural applications. Pyrethroids are discussed separately in Chapter 8.

Toxicology

Crude pyrethrum is a dermal and respiratory allergen, probably due mainly to non-insecticidal ingredients. Contact dermatitis and allergic respiratory reactions (rhinitis and asthma) have occurred following exposures.[13,14] Single cases exhibiting anaphylactic[15] and pneumonitic manifestations[16] have also been reported. The refined pyrethrins are probably less allergenic, but appear to retain some irritant and/or sensitizing properties.

Pyrethrins are absorbed across the gut and pulmonary membrane, but only slightly across intact skin. They are very effectively hydrolyzed to inert products by mammalian liver enzymes. This rapid degradation combined with relatively poor bioavailability probably accounts in large part for their relatively low mammalian toxicity. Dogs fed extraordinary doses exhibit tremor, ataxia, labored breathing, and salivation. Similar neurotoxicity rarely, if ever, has been observed in humans, even in individuals who have used pyrethrins for body lice control (extensive contact) or pyrethrum as an anthelmintic (ingestion).

In cases of human exposure to commercial products, the possible role of other toxicants in the products should be kept in mind. The synergists piperonyl butoxide and n–octyl bicycloheptene dicarboximide have low toxic potential in humans, but organophosphates or carbamates included in the product may have significant toxicity. Pyrethrins themselves do not inhibit cholinesterase enzyme.

Confirmation of Poisoning

There are at present no practical tests for pyrethrin metabolites or pyrethrin effects on human enzymes or tissues that can be used to confirm absorption.

Treatment

1. Antihistamines are effective in controlling most allergic reactions. Severe asthmatic reactions, particularly in predisposed persons, may require administration of inhaled B_2-agonists and/or systemic corticosteroids. Inhalation exposure should be carefully avoided in the future.

2. Anaphylaxis-type reactions may require sub-cutaneous epinephrine, epinepherine, and respiratory support.[15]

3. Contact dermatitis may require extended administration of topical corticosteroid preparations. This should be done under the supervision of a physician. Future contact with the allergen must be avoided.

4. Eye contamination should be removed by flushing the eye with large amounts of clean water or saline. Specialized ophthalmologic care should be obtained if irritation persists.

5. Other toxic manifestations caused by other ingredients must be treated according to their respective toxic actions, independent of pyrethrin-related effects.

6. Gastrointestinal decontamination. Even though most ingestions of pyrethrin products present little risk, if a large amount of pyrethrin-containing material has been ingested and the patient is seen within one hour, consider gastric emptying. If the patient is seen later, or if gastric emptying is performed, consider administration of activated charcoal as described in Chapter 2.

ROTENONE

Although this natural substance is present in a number of plants, the source of most rotenone used in the United States is the dried derris root imported from Central and South America. It is formulated as dusts, powders, and sprays (less than 5% active ingredient) for use in gardens and on food crops. Many products contain piperonyl butoxide as synergist, and other pesticides are included in some commercial products. Rotenone degrades rapidly in the environment. Emulsions of rotenone are applied to lakes and ponds to kill fish.

Toxicology

Although rotenone is toxic to the nervous systems of insects, fish, and birds, commercial rotenone products have presented little hazard to humans over many decades. Neither fatalities nor systemic poisonings have been reported in relation to ordinary use. However, there is one report of a fatality in a child who ingested a product called Gallocide, which contains rotenone and etheral oils, including clove oil. She developed a gradual loss of consciousness over two hours and died of respiratory arrest.[17]

Numbness of oral mucous membranes has been reported in workers who got dust from the powdered derris root in their mouths. Dermatitis and respiratory tract irritation have also been reported in occupationally exposed persons.

When rotenone has been injected into animals, tremors, vomiting, incoordination, convulsions, and respiratory arrest have been observed. These effects have not been reported in occupationally exposed humans.

Treatment

1. Skin decontamination. Skin contamination should be removed by washing with soap and water. Eye contamination should be removed by flushing the eye thoroughly with clean water or saline. Dust in the mouth should be washed out. If irritation persists, medical treatment should be obtained.

2. Gastrointestinal decontamination. If a large amount of a rotenone-containing product has been swallowed and retained and the patient is seen within an hour of exposure, consideration should be given to gastric emptying. Whether or not gastric emptying is performed, consider use of activated charcoal as outlined in Chapter 2.

3. Respiratory support should be used as necessary if mental status changes and/or respiratory depression occurs.

SABADILLA (Veratrum alkaloid)

Sabadilla consists of the powdered ripe seeds of a South American lily. It is used as dust, with lime or sulfur, or dissolved in kerosene, mainly to kill ectoparasites on domestic animals and humans. Insecticidal alkaloids are those of the veratrum type. The concentration of alkaloids in commercial sabadilla is usually less than 0.5%. Little or no sabadilla is used in the United States today, but some is probably used in other countries. Most toxic encounters with veratrum alkaloid occur from the inadvertent ingestion of the plant.[18]

Toxicology

Sabadilla dust is very irritating to the upper respiratory tract, causing sneezing, and is also irritating to the skin. Veratrin alkaloids are apparently absorbed across the skin and gut, and probably by the lung as well. Veratrin alkaloids have a digitalis-like action on the heart muscles (impaired conduction and arrhythmia).

Although poisoning by medicinal veratrum preparations may have occurred in the past, systemic poisoning by sabadilla preparations used as insecticides has been very rare. The prominent symptoms of veratrum alkaloid poisoning are severe nausea and vomiting, followed by hypotension and bradycardia. Other arrythmias or A-V block may occur.[18,19]

Treatment

1. Skin decontamination. Contaminated skin should be washed thoroughly with soap and water. If eyes are affected, they should be flushed with copious amounts of clean water or saline. If skin or eye irritation persists, medical treatment should be obtained.

2. Gastrointestinal decontamination. If a large amount of sabadilla pesticide product has been ingested in the past hour and retained, consider gastric emptying. This may be followed by administration of charcoal. If only a small amount of sabadilla pesticide has been ingested and retained, or if treatment is delayed, and if the patient remains fully alert, immediate oral administration of activated charcoal probably represents reasonable management, as outlined in Chapter 2.

3. Cardiac monitoring. If there is a suspicion that significant amounts of sabadilla alkaloids have been absorbed, ECG monitoring of cardiac activity for arrhythmia and conduction defects is appropriate. Bradycardia may be treated with atropine.[18,19] See dosage on next page.

> **Dosage of Atropine Sulfate:**
>
> - *Adults and children over 12 years:* 0.4-0.5 mg slowly IV, repeated every 5 minutes if necessary.
>
> - *Children under 12 years:* 0.01 mg/kg body weight, slowly IV, repeated every 5 minutes if necessary. (There is a minimum dose of 0.1 mg).

STREPTOMYCIN

Streptomycin sulfate and nitrate are used as pesticides for the control of a variety of commercially important bacterial plant pathogens. Streptomycin is an antibiotic derived from the growth of *Streptomyces griseus*.

Toxicology

This antibiotic shares a toxic profile with the aminoglycoside antibiotics commonly used to treat human diseases. Its major modes of toxicity are nephrotoxicity and ototoxicity. Fortunately, it is poorly absorbed from the gastrointestinal tract, so systemic toxicity is unlikely with ingestion.

Treatment

If a large amount of streptomycin has been ingested within one hour of the patient's receiving care, gastric emptying should be considered. Administration of activated charcoal, as outlined in Chapter 2, should be considered.

References

1. Samples JR and Buettner H. Corneal ulcer caused by a biological insecticide (Bacillus thuringiensis). *Am J Ophthalmol* 1983;95:258.

2. Isaacs G. Permanent local anesthesia and anhydrosis after clove oil spillage. *Lancet* 1983;1:882.

3. Barkin ME, Boyd JP, and Cohen S. Acute allergic reaction to eugenol. *Oral Surg Oral Med Oral Pathol* 1984;57:441-2.

4. Lane BW, Ellenhorn MJ, Hulbert TV, et al. Clove oil ingestion in an infant. *Hum Exp Toxicol* 1991;10:291-4.

5. Hartnoll G, Moore D, and Douek D. Near fatal ingestion of oil of cloves. *Arch Dis Child* 1993;69:392-3.

6. Lavoie FW and Harris TM. Fatal nicotine ingestion. *J Emerg Med* 1991;9:133-6.

7. Svensson CK. Clinical pharmacokinetics of nicotine. *Clin Pharm* 1987;12:30-40.

8. Kyerematen MS, Damiano MD, Dvorchik BH, et al. Smoking-induced changes in nicotine disposition: Application of a new HPLC assay for nicotine and its metabolites. *Clin Pharmacol Ther* 1982;32:769-80.

9. Feyerabend C, Ings RMJ, and Russell MAH. Nicotine pharmacokinetics and its application to intake from smoking. *Br J Clin Pharmacol* 1985;19:239-47.

10. Woolf A, Burkhart K, Caraccio T, et al. Self-poisoning among adults using multiple transdermal nicotine patches. *J Toxicol Clin Toxicol* 1996;34:691-8.

11. Sanchez P, Ducasse JL, Lapeyre-Mestre M, et al. Nicotine poisoning as a cause of cardiac arrest? (letter). *J Toxicol Clin Toxicol* 1996;34:475-6.

12. Malizia E, Andreucci G, Alfani F, et al. Acute intoxication with nicotine alkaloids and cannabinoids in children from ingestion of cigarettes. *Hum Toxicol* 1983;2:315-6.

13. Moretto A. Indoor spraying with the pyrethroid insecticide lambda-cyhalothrin: Effects on spraymen and inhabitants of sprayed houses. *Bull World Health Organ* 1991; 69:591-4.

14. Newton JG and Breslin ABX. Asthmatic reactions to a commonly used aerosol insect killer. *Med J Aust* 1983; 1:378-80.

15. Culver CA, Malina JJ, and Talbert RL. Probable anaphylactoid reaction to a pyrethrin pediculocide shampoo. *Clin Pharm* 1988;7:846-9.

16. Carlson JE and Villaveces JW. Hypersensitivity pneumonitis due to pyrethrum. *JAMA* 1977;237:1718-9.

17. DeWilde AR. A case of fatal rotenone poisoning in a child. *J Forensic Sci* 1986;31(4):1492-8.

18. Jaffe AM, Gephardt D, and Courtemanche L. Poisoning due to ingestion of veratrum viride (false hellebore). *J Emerg Med* 1990;8:161-7.

19. Quatrehomme G, Bertrand F, Chauvet C, et al. Intoxication from veratrum album. *Hum Exp Toxicol* 1993;12:111-5.

CHAPTER 8

Other Insecticides, Acaricides, and Repellents

This chapter discusses insecticides, acaricides, and repellents that have toxicologic characteristics distinct from the insecticides discussed in previous chapters. Pesticides reviewed include: alkyl phthalates, benzyl benzoate, borates, chlordimeform, chlorobenzilate, cyhexatin, diethyltoluamide, fluorides, haloaromatic urea compounds, methoprene, propargite, pyrethroids, and sulfur.

ALKYL PHTHALATES

Dimethyl phthalate has been widely used as an insect repellent applied directly to the skin. Dibutylphthalate is impregnated into fabric for the same purpose. It is more resistant to laundering than dimethyl phthalate.

Toxicology

Dimethyl phthalate is strongly irritating to the eyes and mucous membranes. It has caused little or no irritation when applied to skin, and dermal absorption is apparently minimal. It has not caused sensitization. Tests in rodents have indicated low systemic toxicity, but large ingested doses cause gastrointestinal irritation, central nervous system depression, coma, and hypotension.

Treatment

No antidote is available. Supportive measures (hydration, oxygen if needed) are probably adequate to manage all but the most severe poisonings.

BENZYL BENZOATE

Toxicology

Incorporated into lotions and ointments, this agent has been used for many years in veterinary and human medicine against mites and lice. Apart from occasional cases of skin irritation, adverse effects have been few. The efficiency of skin absorption is not known. Absorbed benzyl benzoate is rapidly biotransformed to hippuric acid which is excreted in the urine. When given in large doses to laboratory animals, benzyl benzoate causes excitement, incoordination, paralysis of the limbs, convulsions, respiratory paralysis, and death. No human poisonings have been reported.

Treatment

1. Skin decontamination. If significant irritant effect appears, medications should be discontinued and the skin cleansed with soap and water. Eye contamination should be treated by prolonged flushing with clean water or saline.

2. Gastrointestinal decontamination. If a potentially toxic amount has been swallowed and retained and the patient is seen soon after exposure, gastrointestinal decontamination should be considered as outlined in Chapter 2.

3. Seizures. If seizures occur, control may require anticonvulsant medication as outlined in Chapter 2.

BORIC ACID AND BORATES

Boric acid is formulated as tablets and powder to kill larvae in livestock confinement areas and cockroaches, ants, and other insects in residences. Rarely, solutions are sprayed as a nonselective herbicide.

Toxicology

Boric acid powders and pellets scattered on the floors of homes do present a hazard to children. Their frequent use for roach control increases access for ingestion. A series of 784 patients has been described with no fatalities and minimum toxicity. Only 12% of these patients had symptoms of toxicity, mostly to the gastrointestinal tract.[1] However, there have been some recent reports of fatal poisonings,[2,3] and a great many poisonings of newborns which occurred in the 1950s and 1960s often ended in death.[4,5] Historically, many poisonings have resulted from injudicious uses in human medicine aimed at suppressing bacterial growth, such as compresses for burns, powders for diaper rash, and irrigation solutions.[6,7] With the increased use of boric acid for roach control, suicidal or accidental ingestion is still likely to occur.[3,7]

Borax dust is moderately irritating to skin. Inhaled dust caused irritation of the respiratory tract among workers in a borax plant. Symptoms included nasal irritation, mucous membrane dryness, cough, shortness of breath, and chest tightness.[8,9]

Commercial Products

ALKYL PHTHALATES

dibutylphthalate
dimethyl phthalate
DMP

BENZYL BENZOATE

BORIC ACID AND BORATES

boric acid
sodium polyborates
Polybor 3
sodium tetraborate decahydrate
Borax

CHLORDIMEFORM (nr)

CHLOROBENZILATE (nr)

Acaraben
Akar
Benzilan
Folbex

CYHEXATIN (nr)

Acarstin
Metaran
Oxotin
Pennstyl
Plictran

DIETHYLTOLUAMIDE (DEET)

Auton
Detamide
Metadelphene
MGK
Muskol
Off!
Skeeter Beater
Skeeter Cheater
Skintastic for Kids

FLUORIDES

sodium fluoride (wood protection only)
sodium fluosilicate (sodium silico fluoride) (nr)
Prodan
Safsan
sodium fluoaluminate
Cryolite
Kryocide
Prokil

(Continued on the next page)

When determining toxicity to boric acid from ingestion, it is important to distinguish between acute and chronic exposure. Chronic ingestion is more likely to cause significant toxicity than acute exposure.[1,2] Borates are well absorbed by the gut and by abraded or burned skin, but not by intact skin.[6] The kidney efficiently excretes them. The residence half-life in humans averages 13 hours, in a range of 4-28 hours.[1]

The gastrointestinal tract, skin, vascular system, and brain are the principal organs and tissues effected. Nausea, persistent vomiting, abdominal pain, and diarrhea reflect a toxic gastroenteritis.[1,2,7] Lethargy and headache may occur, but are more infrequent.[1] In severe poisonings, a beefy red skin rash, most often affecting palms, soles, buttocks, and scrotum, has been described. It has been characterized as a "boiled lobster appearance." The intense erythema is followed by extensive exfoliation.[2,5,10] This may be difficult to distinguish from staphylcoccal scalded skin syndrome.[10]

Headache, weakness, lethargy, restlessness, and tremors may occur, but are less frequent than gastrointestinal effects.[1] Seven infants who were exposed to a mixture of borax and honey on their pacifiers developed seizures.[11] Unconsciousness and respiratory depression signify life-threatening brain injury. Cyanosis, weak pulse, hypotension, and cold clammy skin indicate shock, which is sometimes the cause of death in borate poisoning.[2,3,7]

Acute renal failure (oliguria or anuria) may be a consequence of shock, of direct toxic action on renal tubule cells, or both. It occurs in severe borate poisoning.[2,3,5,10] Metabolic acidosis may be a consequence of the acid itself, of seizure activity, or of metabolic derangements.[2] Fever is sometimes present in the absence of infection.

Confirmation of Poisoning

Borate can be measured in serum by colorimetric methods, as well by high-temperature atomic spectrometric methods. Urine borate concentrations in non-exposed individuals are in the range of 0.004-.66 mg/dL. Normal serum levels range up to 0.2 mg/dL in adults, and in children to 0.125 mg/dL.[7] Levels reported in toxic incidents have varied widely, and it is felt that serum levels are of little use in guiding therapy.[1]

Treatment

1. Skin decontamination. Wash skin with soap and water as outlined in Chapter 2. Eye contamination should be removed by prolonged flushing of the eye with copious amounts of clean water or saline. If irritation persists, specialized medical treatment should be obtained.

2. Gastrointestinal decontamination. In acute poisonings, if a large amount has been ingested and the patient is seen within one hour of exposure, gastrointestinal decontamination should be considered as outlined in Chapter 2. It is important to keep in mind that vomiting and diarrhea are common, and severe poisoning may be associated with seizures. Therefore induction of emesis by syrup of ipecac is probably contraindicated in these exposures. Catharsis is not indicated if diarrhea is present.

3. Intravenous fluids. If ingestion of borate has been massive (several grams), or has extended over several days, administer intravenous glucose and electrolyte solutions to sustain urinary excretion of borate. Monitor fluid balance and serum electrolytes (including bicarbonate capacity) regularly. Monitor cardiac status by ECG. Test the urine for protein and cells to detect renal injury, and monitor serum concentration of borate. Metabolic acidosis may be treated with sodium bicarbonate. If shock develops, it may be necessary to infuse plasma or whole blood. Administer oxygen continuously. If oliguria (less than 25–30 mL urine formed per hour) occurs, intravenous fluids must be slowed or stopped to avoid overloading the circulation. Such patients should usually be referred to a center capable of providing intensive care for critically ill patients.

4. Hemodialysis. If renal failure occurs, hemodialysis may be necessary to sustain fluid balance and normal extracellular fluid composition. Hemodialysis has had limited success in enhancing clearance of borates.[1]

5. Peritoneal dialysis has been performed in borate poisoning[5,12] and is felt to be as effective as, and safer than, exchange transfusion in removing borate. No large study of efficacy has been done, but it is still used somewhat less frequently than hemodialysis.[1]

6. Seizures should be controlled as recommended for other agents and outlined Chapter 2.

CHLORDIMEFORM

Chlordimeform is an ovicide and acaricide. Formulations are emulsifiable concentrates and water-soluble powders.

Toxicology

In a reported episode of occupational exposure to chlordimeform, several workers developed hematuria. Hemorrhagic cystitis, probably due to chloraniline biodegradation products, was the source of the blood in the urine. Symptoms reported by the affected workers included gross hematuria, dysuria, urinary frequency and urgency, penile discharge, abdominal and back pain, a general-

Commercial Products

(Continued)

Demon
Flectron
Folcord
KafilSuper
NRDC 149
Polytrin
Ripcord
Siperin
Ustadd
others
deltamethrin
  Decis
  DeltaDust
  DeltaGard
  Deltex
  Suspend
dimethrin
fenothrin (nr)
fenpropanate (nr)
fenpropathrin
  Danitol
  Herald
  Meothrin
  Rody
fenvalerate
  Belmark
  Fenkill
  Sumicidin
flucythrinate
  Cybolt
  Fluent
  Payoff
fluvalinate
furethrin (nr)
permethrin
  Ambush
  Dragnet
  Eksmin
  Elimite
  Kafil
  Nix
  Outflank
  Permasect
  Perthrine
  Pounce
  Pramex
  Talcord
  others
phthalthrin (nr)
resmethrin
  Benzofuroline
  Chrysron
  Pynosect

(Continued on the next page)

tetramethrin
  Neopynamin
tralomethrin
  SAGA
  Tralex

SULFUR

  many commercial products

nr = not registered or withdrawn

ized "hot" sensation, sleepiness, skin rash and desquamation, a sweet taste, and anorexia. Symptoms persisted for 2-8 weeks after exposure was terminated.[13] In a single case, methemoglobinemia was reported.[14] Chlordimeform is not a cholinesterase inhibitor. Chlordimeform has been voluntarily cancelled in the U.S. due to concerns regarding increased bladder cancer incidence seen in manufacturing workers.

Confirmation of Poisoning

Although methods do exist for measurement of urinary excretion products, these tests are not generally available.

Treatment

1. Precautions. Strenuous efforts should be made to protect against inhalation and dermal contact with chlordimeform because absorption is evidently efficient.

2. Skin decontamination. Wash skin with soap and water as outlined in Chapter 2. Eye contamination should be removed by prolonged flushing of the eye with copious amounts of clean water or saline. If irritation persists, specialized medical treatment should be obtained.

3. Gastrointestinal decontamination. If chlordimeform has been ingested no more than an hour prior to treatment, consider gastrointestinal decontamination as outlined in Chapter 2. Repeated doses of charcoal every 2-4 hours may be beneficial.

4. Hydration. Because catharsis may cause serious dehydration and electrolyte disturbances in young children, fluid balance and serum electrolytes should be monitored. An adequate state of hydration should be maintained by oral and/or intravenous fluids to support chlordimeform excretion.

5. Urinary analysis. Repeated analyses of urine for protein and red cells should be done to detect injury to the urinary tract. Disappearance of hematuria can ordinarily be expected in 2-8 weeks. Relief from other symptoms can usually be expected earlier.

CHLOROBENZILATE

Chlorobenzilate is a chlorinated hydrocarbon acaricide, usually formulated as an emulsion or wettable powder for application in orchards. Use in the United States has been discontinued.

Toxicology

Chlorobenzilate is moderately irritating to the skin and eyes. Although structurally similar to DDT, chlorobenzilate is much more rapidly excreted following absorption, chiefly in the urine as the benzophenone and benzoic acid derivatives. Based on observation of dosed animals, extreme absorbed doses may cause tremors, ataxia, and muscle weakness. There has been one case in humans of toxic encephalopathy following spraying in a field for 14 days at 10 hours per day. The patient did not wear a mask while spraying. His symptoms included muscle pain, weakness, fever, and mental status changes progressing to a tonic–clonic seizure. He recovered without sequelae within 6 days. Treatment included respiratory support and seizure control with phenobarbital and phenytoin.[15]

Chlorobenzilate is not a cholinesterase inhibitor.

Treatment

1. Skin decontamination. Wash skin with soap and water as outlined in Chapter 2. Eye contamination should be removed by prolonged flushing of the eye with copious amounts of clean water or saline. If irritation persists, specialized medical treatment should be obtained.

2. Gastrointestinal decontamination. If a large amount of chlorobenzilate was ingested within a few hours prior to treatment, consider gastrointestinal decontamination as outlined in Chapter 2. If the absorbed dose of chlorobenzilate was small, if treatment is delayed, and if the patient is asymptomatic, oral administration of activated charcoal and sorbitol may be indicated. Do not give fats or oils.

3. Seizures. Any seizures should be treated as outlined in Chapter 2.

CYHEXATIN

Toxicology

Tricyclohexyl tin hydroxide is formulated as a 50% wettable powder for control of mites on ornamentals, hops, nut trees, and some fruit trees. It is moderately irritating, particularly to the eyes. While information on the systemic toxicity of this specific tin compound is lacking, it should probably be assumed that cyhexatin can be absorbed to some extent across the skin, and that substantial absorbed doses would cause nervous system injury (see organotin compounds in Chapter 15, Fungicides). Cyhexatin has been voluntarily cancelled in the United States.

Treatment

1. Skin decontamination. Wash skin with soap and water. Remove contamination from the eyes by prolonged flushing with clean water or saline.

2. Gastrointestinal decontamination. Management of poisonings by ingestion should proceed on the assumption that cyhexatin is toxic, even though rodent LD_{50} values are fairly high, and no human poisonings have been reported. Treatment should be as with other organotin compounds.

DIETHYLTOLUAMIDE (DEET)

This chemical is a widely-used liquid insect repellent, suitable for application to skin or to fabrics. It comes in a wide range of concentrations from 5% (Off!, Skintastic for Kids[R]) to 100% (Muskol[R]). Compared to the widespread use of the product, there are relatively few cases of toxicity.[16] However, if used improperly, ingested, or a very high concentration is used on children, especially repeatedly over large skin surfaces, the potential for severe toxicity exists.[17] DEET is formulated with ethyl or isopropyl alcohol.

Toxicology

For many years, diethyltoluamide has been effective and generally well tolerated as an insect repellent applied to human skin, although tingling, mild irritation, and sometimes desquamation have followed repeated application. In some cases, DEET has caused contact dermatitis and excerbation of pre-existing skin disease.[18,19] It is very irritating to the eyes, but not corrosive.

Serious adverse effects have occurred when used under tropical condition, when it was applied to areas of skin that were occluded during sleep (mainly the antecubital and popliteal fossae). Under these conditions, the skin became red and tender, then exhibited blistering and erosion, leaving painful weeping denuded areas that were slow to heal. Severe scarring occasionally resulted from some of these severe reactions.[20]

DEET is efficiently absorbed across the skin and by the gut. Blood concentrations of about 0.3 mg/dL have been reported several hours after dermal application in the prescribed fashion.[17] The amount absorbed increases as the concentration of DEET rises. In addition, many commercial formulations are prepared with ethanol as a solvent, which further increases absorption.[21] Toxic encephalopathic reactions have apparently occurred in rare instances following dermal application, mainly in children who were intensively treated.[22, 23,24] The more frequent cause of systemic toxicity has been ingestion: deliberate in adults and accidental in young children.[16,17]

Manifestations of toxic encephalopathy have been behavioral disorders including headache, restlessness, irritability, ataxia, rapid loss of consciousness, hypotension, and seizures. Some cases have shown flaccid paralysis and areflexia. Deaths have occurred following very large doses.[16,17,22] Blood levels of DEET found in fatal systemic poisonings have ranged from 168 to 240 mg per liter.[17] Interpretation of DEET toxicity in some fatal cases has been complicated by effects of simultaneously ingested ethanol, tranquilizers, and other drugs. One well-documented case of anaphylactic reaction to DEET has been reported. One fatal case of encephalopathy in a child heterozygous for ornithine carbamoyl transferase deficiency resembled Reyes syndrome, but the postmortem appearance of the liver was not characteristic of the syndrome.

Discretion should be exercised in recommending DEET for persons who have acne, psoriasis, an atopic predisposition, or other chronic skin condition. It should not be applied to any skin area that is likely to be opposed to another skin surface for a significant period of time (antecubital and popliteal fossae, inguinal areas).[22]

Great caution should be exercised in using DEET on children. Avoid repeated application day after day. Applications should be limited to exposed areas of skin, using as little repellent as possible and washing off after use. Do not apply to eyes and mouth and, with young children, do not apply to their hands. Low concentrations (10% or below) are effective and may be preferred in most situations. There are formulations labeled for children that have concentrations of 5 to 6.5% DEET.[25] If continuous repellent protection is necessary, DEET should be alternated with a repellent having another active ingredient. If headache or any kind of emotional or behavioral change occurs, use of DEET should be discontinued immediately.

Confirmation of Poisoning

Methods exist for measurement of DEET in blood and tissues and of metabolites in urine, but these are not widely available.

Treatment

1. Skin decontamination. Wash skin with soap and water as outlined in Chapter 2. Eye contamination should be removed by prolonged flushing of the eye with copious amounts of clean water or saline. If irritation persists, specialized medical treatment should be obtained. Topical steroids and oral antihistamines have been used for severe skin reactions that occasionally follow application of DEET.[21]

2. Gastrointestinal decontamination. If a substantial amount of DEET has been ingested within an hour of treatment, gastrointestinal decontamination should be considered as outlined in Chapter 2. Induced emesis is usually considered contraindicated in these poisonings due to the rapid onset of seizures.

3. Seizures. Treatment is primarily supportive, with control of seizures by anticonvulsants, as outlined in Chapter 2. Persons surviving poisoning by ingestion of DEET have usually recovered within 36 hours or less.[16,17]

FLUORIDES

Sodium fluoride is a crystalline mineral once widely used in the United States for control of larvae and crawling insects in homes, barns, warehouses, and other storage areas. It is highly toxic to all plant and animal life. The only remaining use permitted is for wood treatement

Sodium fluosilicate (sodium silico fluoride) has been used to control ectoparasites on livestock, as well as crawling insects in homes and work buildings. It is approximately as toxic as sodium fluoride. All uses in the U.S. have been cancelled.

Sodium fluoaluminate (Cryolite) is a stable mineral containing fluoride. It is used as an insecticide on some vegetables and fruits. Cryolite has very low water solubility, does not yield fluoride ion on decomposition, and presents very little toxic hazard to mammals, including humans.

Hydrofluoric acid is an important industrial toxicant, but is not used as a pesticide. Sulfuryl fluoride is discussed in Chapter 16, Fumigants.

Toxicology

Sodium fluoride and fluosilicate used as insecticides present a serious hazard to humans because of high inherent toxicity, and the possibility that children crawling on floors of treated dwellings will ingest the material.

Absorption across the skin is probably slight, and methods of pesticide use rarely include a hazard of inhalation, but uptake of ingested fluoride by the gut is efficient and potentially lethal. Excretion is chiefly in the urine. Within the first 24 hours of intoxication, renal clearance of fluoride from the blood is rapid. However, patients go on to continue to excrete large amounts of fluoride for several days. This is thought to be due to a rapid binding of fluoride to a body store, probably bone. The subsequent release of fluoride from bone is gradual enough not to cause a recurrence of toxicity.[26, 27] Large loads of absorbed fluoride may potentially poison renal tubule cells, resulting in acute renal failure. Children will have greater skeletal uptake of fluoride than adults, therefore limiting the amount the kidney needs to handle. Despite this, children are still at great risk because of their smaller body mass compared to adults in relation to the amount ingested.[27]

The toxic effects of fluoride in mammals are multiple, and all may threaten life. The primary effects from fluoride result from an inhibition of critical intra-cellular enzymes and the direct effect on ionized calcium in extra–cellular fluid. Hypocalcemia commonly occurs.[26, 28,29, 30]

Ingested fluoride is transformed in the stomach to hydrofluoric acid, which has a corrosive effect on the epithelial lining of the gastrointestinal tract. Thirst, abdominal pain, vomiting, and diarrhea are usual symptoms. Hemorrhage in the gastric mucosa, ulceration, erosions, and edema are common signs.[31]

Absorbed fluoride ion reduces extracellular fluid concentrations of calcium and magnesium. Hypocalcemia sometimes results in tetany.[30] Cardiac arrhythmia and shock are often prominent features of severe poisoning. Hypotension and severe arrhythmia, sometimes progressing to ventricular fibrillation, may also occur.[26, 32] These probably result from combinations of effects of fluid and electrolyte disturbances including hyperkalemia[32] and direct actions of fluoride on heart and vascular tissues. Fluoride may directly affect the central nervous system, resulting in headache, muscle weakness, stupor, convulsions, and coma.[26,27,28] Respiratory failure and ventricular arrythmias are common causes of death.[26,27]

Confirmation of Poisoning

A population drinking water with a concentration of 1 mg per liter will have a plasma inorganic fluoride concentration between 0.01 and 0.03 mg per liter[28] and rarely above 0.10 mg per liter. In fatal cases of poisoning, plasma levels of 3.5 mg per liter and higher have been recorded, although survival has been reported in patients with levels as high as 14 mg per liter.[26,28]

Treatment: Fluoride Toxicosis

1. Skin decontamination. Wash skin with soap and water as outlined in Chapter 2. Eye contamination should be removed by prolonged flushing of the eye with copious amounts of clean water or saline. If irritation persists, specialized medical treatment should be obtained.

2. Gastrointestinal decontamination. If **sodium fluoride or sodium fluosilicate** has been ingested, consider gastric decontamination as outlined in Chapter 2.

If the victim is obtunded or if vomiting precludes oral administration, the airway should be protected by endotracheal intubation, then the stomach should be gently intubated and lavaged with several ounces of one of the liquids named below. Activated charcoal is not likely to be of use because it does not bind the fluoride ion well.

3. Calcium and magnesium. If the victim is fully alert, and if vomiting does not totally prevent swallowing of a neutralizing agent, prompt oral administration of **milk, calcium gluconate, or magnesium citrate** will precipitate fluoride ion in the gut and therefore may be life-saving. The milk provides the calcium ions that will bind to fluoride, thereby reducing absorption. Magnesium–based antacids have also been used to neutralize the acid and facilitate the production of poorly absorbed salts.[26] There are no data on the optimum amounts to be administered.

4. Blood analysis. A blood specimen should be drawn for serum electrolyte analysis for sodium, potassium, calcium, magnesium, fluoride, and bicarbonate capacity. Blood should also be drawn to type and cross match for blood transfusion.

5. Intravenous fluids (initially 5% dextrose in 0.9% saline) should be started to combat dehydration, shock, and metabolic acidosis. Fluid balance should be monitored closely to forestall fluid overload if renal failure occurs. If metabolic acidosis is detected, sodium bicarbonate should be administered to keep the urine alkaline as this may hasten excretion.[27] Intravenous fluids must be stopped if anuria or oliguria (less than 25–30 mL per hour) develops.

6. Hemodialysis should be reserved for compromised renal function.[26]

7. Monitor cardiac status by continuous electrocardiography. Ventricular arrhythmia may necessitate DC cardioversion.

8. Tetany. If overt or latent tetany occurs, or if hypocalcemia is demonstrated, or if it appears likely that a significant amount of fluoride has been absorbed, administer 10 mL of 10% **calcium gluconate** intravenously, at no more than 1 mL per minute.

Dosage of Calcium Gluconate:
Supplied as 100 mg/mL (10% solution)

- *Adults and children over 12 years:* 10 mL of 10% solution, given slowly, intravenously. Repeat as necessary.

- *Children under 12 years:* 200–500 mg/kg/24 hr divided Q6 hr. For cardiac arrest, 100 mg/kg/dose. Repeat dosage as needed.

---

9. Oxygen by mask should be administered for hypotension, shock, cardiac arrhythmia, or cyanosis. Shock may require administration of plasma or blood.

10. Acid Burns. Since these compounds can cause severe acid burns to the esophagus and stomach, patients should be referred for surgical evaluation and endoscopy. If burns are documented, treatment for acid burns should be continued by a surgeon or gastroenterologist.

Treatment: Sodium Fluoaluminate (Cryolite)

Cryolite is much less toxic than other fluorides. If a very large amount has been ingested, it may be appropriate to measure serum calcium to insure that hypocalcemia has not occurred. If so, intravenous 10% calcium gluconate would be indicated (see 8 above). It is unlikely that treatment for fluoride toxicity would be necessary following ingestion of sodium fluoaluminate.

HALOAROMATIC SUBSTITUTED UREAS

Diflubenzuron is a haloaromatic substituted urea which controls insects by impairing chitin deposition in the larval exoskeleton. It is formulated in wettable powders, oil dispersible concentrate, and granules for use in agriculture and forestry, for aerial application against gypsy moth, and in settings where fly populations tend to be large, such as feedlots. Teflubenzuron is another haloaromatic substituted urea insecticide with similar toxicologic properties.

Toxicology

There is limited absorption of diflubenzuron across the skin and intestinal lining of mammals, after which enzymatic hydrolysis and excretion rapidly eliminate the pesticide from tissues. Irritant effects are not reported and systemic toxicity is low. Methemoglobinemia is a theoretical risk from chloraniline formed hydrolytically, but no reports of this form of toxicity have been reported in humans or animals from diflubenzuron exposure. Teflubenzuron also shows low systemic toxicity.

Treatment

1. Skin decontamination. Wash skin with soap and water as outlined in Chapter 2. Eye contamination should be removed by prolonged flushing of the eye with copious amounts of clean water or saline. If irritation persists, obtain specialized medical treatment. Sensitization reactions may require steroid therapy.

2. Gastrointestinal decontamination. If large amounts of propargite have been ingested and the patient is seen within an hour, consider gastrointestinal decontamination. For small ingestions, consider oral administration of activated charcoal and sorbitol.

METHOPRENE

Methoprene is a long chain hydrocarbon ester active as an insect growth regulator. It is effective against several insect species. Formulations include slow-release briquets, sprays, foggers, and baits.

Toxicology

Methoprene is neither an irritant nor a sensitizer in humans or laboratory animals. Systemic toxicity in laboratory animals is very low. No human poisonings or adverse reactions in exposed workers have been reported.

Treatment

1. Skin decontamination. Wash contaminated skin with soap and water. Flush contamination from eyes with copious amounts of clean water or saline. If irritation persists, medical attention must be obtained.

2. Gastrointestinal decontamination. If a very large amount of methoprene has been ingested, oral administration of charcoal may be considered.

PROPARGITE

Propargite is an acaricide with residual action. Formulations are wettable powders and emulsifiable concentrates.

Toxicology

Propargite exhibits very little systemic toxicity in animals. No systemic poisonings have been reported in humans. However, many workers having dermal contact with this acaricide, especially during the summer months, have experienced skin irritation and possibly sensitization in some cases.[33] Eye irritation has also occurred. For this reason, stringent measures should be taken to prevent inhalation or any skin or eye contamination by propargite.

Confirmation of Poisoning

There is no readily available method for detecting absorption of propargite.

Treatment

Treatment of contamination and ingestions should proceed essentially as outlined for haloaromatic substituted urea.

PYRETHROIDS

These modern synthetic insecticides are similar chemically to natural pyrethrins, but modified to increase stability in the natural environment. They are now widely used in agriculture, in homes and gardens, and for treatment of ectoparasitic disease.

Pyrethroids are formulated as emulsifiable concentrates, wettable powders, granules, and concentrates for ultra low volume application. They may be combined with additional pesticides (sometimes highly toxic) in the technical product or tank-mixed with other pesticides at the time of application. AASTAR (discontinued 1992), for instance, was a combination of flucythrinate and phorate. Phorate is a highly toxic organophosphate. Nix and Elimite are permethrin creams applied to control human ectoparasites.

Toxicology

Certain pyrethroids exhibit striking neurotoxicity in laboratory animals when administered by intravenous injection, and some are toxic by the oral route. However, systemic toxicity by inhalation and dermal absorption is low. Although limited absorption may account for the low toxicity of some pyrethroids, rapid biodegradation by mammalian liver enzymes (ester hydrolysis and oxidation) is probably the major factor responsible for this phenomenon.[34] Most pyrethroid metabolites are promptly excreted, at least in part, by the kidney.

The most severe, although more uncommon, toxicity is to the central nervous system. Seizures have been reported in severe cases of pyrethroid intoxication. Of 573 cases reviewed in China, there were 51 cases with disturbed consciousness and 34 cases with seizures. Of those, only 5 were from occupational exposure.[35] Seizures are more common with exposure to the more toxic cyano-pyrethroids, which include fenvalerate, flucythrinate, cypermethrin, deltapermethrin, and fluvalinate.[34] There are no reports in the literature of seizures in humans from exposure to permethrin.

Apart from central nervous system toxicity, some pyrethroids do cause distressing paresthesias when liquid or volatilized materials contact human skin. Again, these symptoms are more common with exposure to the pyrethroids whose structures include cyano-groups.[34] Sensations are described as stinging, burning, itching, and tingling, progressing to numbness.[35, 36,37] The skin of the face seems to be most commonly affected, but the face, hands, forearms, and neck are sometimes involved. Sweating, exposure to sun or heat, and application of water enhance the disagreeable sensations. Sometimes the effect is noted within minutes of exposure, but a 1-2 hour delay in appearance of symptoms is more common.[36, 37] Sensations rarely persist more than 24 hours. Little or no inflammatory reaction is apparent where the paresthesia are reported; the effect is presumed to result from pyrethroid contact with sensory nerve endings in the skin. The paresthetic reaction is not allergic in nature, although sensitization and allergic responses have been reported as an independent phenomenon with pyrethroid exposure. Neither race, skin type, nor disposition to allergic disease affects the likelihood or severity of the reaction.

Persons treated with permethrin for lice or flea infestations sometimes experience itching and burning at the site of application, but this is chiefly an exacerbation of sensations caused by the parasites themselves, and is not typical of the paresthetic reaction described above.

Other signs and symptoms of toxicity include abnormal facial sensation, dizziness, salivation, headache, fatigue, vomiting, diarrhea, and irritability to sound and touch. In more severe cases, pulmonary edema and muscle fasciculations can develop.[35] Due to the inclusion of unique solvent ingredients, certain formulations of fluvalinate are corrosive to the eyes. Pyrethroids are not cholinesterase inhibitors. However, there have been some cases in which pyrethroid poisoning has been misdiagnosed as organophosphate poisoning, due to some of the similar presenting signs, and some patients have died from atropine toxicity.[35]

Treatment

1. Skin decontamination. Wash skin promptly with soap and water as outlined in Chapter 2. If irritant or paresthetic effects occur, obtain treatment by a physician. Because volatilization of pyrethroids apparently accounts for paresthesia affecting the face, strenuous measures should be taken (ventilation, protective face mask and hood) to avoid vapor contact with the face and eyes. Vitamin E oil preparations (dL–alpha tocopheryl acetate) are uniquely effective in preventing and stopping the paresthetic reaction.[37, 38] They are safe for application to the skin under field conditions. Corn oil is somewhat effective, but possible side effects with continuing use make it less suitable. Vaseline is less effective than corn oil. Zinc oxide actually worsens the reaction.

2. Eye contamination. Some pyrethroid compounds can be very corrosive to the eyes. Extraordinary measures should be taken to avoid eye contamination. The eye should be treated immediately by prolonged flushing of the eye with copious amounts of clean water or saline. If irritation persists, obtain professional ophthalmologic care.

3. Gastrointestinal decontamination. If large amounts of pyrethroids, especially the cyano-pyrethroids, have been ingested and the patient is seen soon after exposure, consider gastrointestinal decontamination as outlined in Chapter 2. Based on observations in laboratory animals[34] and humans,[35] large ingestions of allethrin, cismethrin, fluvalinate, fenvalerate, or deltamethrin would be the most likely to generate neurotoxic manifestations.

If only small amounts of pyrethroid have been ingested, or if treatment has been delayed, oral administration of activated charcoal and cathartic probably represents optimal management. Do not give cathartic if patient has diarrhea or an ileus.

4. Other treatments. Several drugs are effective in relieving the pyrethroid neurotoxic manifestations observed in deliberately poisoned laboratory animals, but none has been tested in human poisonings. Therefore, neither efficacy nor safety under these circumstances is known. Furthermore, moderate neurotoxic symptoms and signs are likely to resolve spontaneously if they do occur.

5. Seizures. Any seizures should be treated as outlined in Chapter 2.

SULFUR

Elemental sulfur is an acaricide and fungicide widely used on orchard, ornamental, vegetable, grain, and other crops. It is prepared as dust in various particle sizes and applied as such, or it may be formulated with various minerals to improve flowability, or applied as an aqueous emulsion or wettable powder.

Toxicology

Elemental sulfur is moderately irritating to the skin and is associated with occupationally related irritant dermatitis.[39] Airborne dust is irritating to the eyes and the respiratory tract. In hot sunny environments, there may be some oxidation of foliage-deposited sulfur to gaseous sulfur oxides, which are very irritating to the eyes and respiratory tract.

Ingested sulfur powder induces catharsis, and has been used medicinally (usually with molasses) for that purpose. Some hydrogen sulfide is formed in the large intestine and this may present a degree of toxic hazard. The characteristic smell of rotten eggs may aid in the diagnosis. An adult has survived ingestion of 200 grams.[40]

Ingested colloidal sulfur is efficiently absorbed by the gut and is promptly excreted in the urine as inorganic sulfate.

Treatment

1. Skin decontamination. Wash skin with soap and water. Contamination of the eyes should be removed by prolonged flushing with clean saline or water. If eye irritation persists, obtain ophthamologic care.

2. Gastrointestinal decontamination. Unless an extraordinary amount of sulfur (several grams) has been ingested shortly prior to treatment, there is probably no need for gastrointestinal decontamination. Adsorbability of sulfur on activated charcoal has not been tested.

The most serious consequence of sulfur ingestion is likely to be that of catharsis, resulting in dehydration and electrolyte depletion, particularly in children. If diarrhea is severe, oral or intravenous administration of glucose and/or electrolyte solutions may be appropriate.

References

1. Litovitz TL, Klein-Schwartz W, Oderda GM, and Schmitz BF. Clinical manifestations of toxicity in a series of 784 boric acid ingestions. *Am J Emerg Med* 1988;6(3):209- 13.

2. Restuccio A, Mortensen ME, and Kelley MT. Fatal ingestion of boric acid in an adult. *Am J Emerg Med* 1992;10(6):545-7.

3. Ishii Y, Fujizuka N, Takahashi T, et al. A fatal case of acute boric acid poisoning. *Clin Toxicol* 1993;31(2):345- 52.

4. Goldbloom RB and Goldbloom A. Boric acid poisoning. *J Pediatr* 1953; 43(6):631- 43.

5. Wong LC, Heimbach MD, Truscott DR, and Duncan BD. Boric acid poisoning. *Can Med Assoc J* 1964;90:1018-23.

6. Ducey J and Williams DB. Transcutaneous absorption of boric acid. *J Pediatr* 1953;43(6):644-51.

7. Linden CH, Hall AH, Kulig KW, and Rumack BH. Acute ingestions of boric acid. *Clin Toxicol* 1986;24(4):269-79.

8. Hu X, Wegman DG, Eisen EA, et al. Dose related acute irritant symptom responses to occupational exposure to sodium borate dusts. *Br J Ind Med* 1992;49:706-13.

9. Garabrant DH, Bernstein L, Peters JM, et al. Respiratory effects of borax dust. *Br J Ind Med* 1985;42:831-7.

10. Schillinger BM, Berstein M, Goldbert LA, and Shalita AR. Boric acid poisoning. *J Am Acad Dermatol* 1982;7(5):667-73.

11. O'Sullivan K and Taylor M. Chronic boric acid poisoning in infants. *Arch Dis Child* 1983;58:737-49.

12. Segar WE. Peritoneal dialysis in the treatment of boric acid poisoning. *New Engl J Med,* 1960;262(16):798-800.

13. Folland DS, Kimbrough RD, Cline RE, et al. Acute hemorrhagic cystitis. *JAMA* 1978;239(11):1052-5.

14. Arima T, Morooka H, Tanigawa T, et al. Methemoglobinemia induced by chlorphenamidine. *Acta Med Okayama* 1976;30:57-60.

15. Ravindran M. Toxic encephalopathy from chlorobenzilate poisoning: Report of a case. *Clin Electroencephalogr* 1978;9(4):170-2.

16. Veltri JC, Osimitz TG, Bradford DC, et al. Retrospective analysis of calls to poison control centers resulting from exposure to the insect repellent N, N-diethyltoluamide (DEET) from 1985-1989. *Clin Toxicol* 1994;32:1.

17. Tenebein M. Severe toxic reactions and death following ingestion of diethyltoluamide-containing insect repellents. *JAMA* 1987;258:1509.

18. Maibach HI and Johnson HL. Contact urticaria syndrome. *Arch Dermatol* 1975;111:726.

19. Wantke F, Focke M, Hemmer W, et al. Generalized urticaria induced by a diethyltoluamide-containing insect repellent in a child. *Contact Dermatitis* 1996;35(3):186.

20. Reuveni H. and Yagupsky P. Diethyltoluamide-containing insect repellent: Adverse effects in worldwide use. *Arch Dermatol* 1982;118:582.

21. Stinecipher J and Shaw J. Percutaneous permeation of N,N-diethyl-m-toluamide (DEET) from commercial mosquito repellents and the effect of solvent. *J Toxicol Environ Health* 1997;52:119.

22. Lipscomb JW, Kramer JE, and Leikin JB. Seizure following brief exposure to the insect repellent N,N-diethyl-m-toluamide. *Ann Emerg Med* 1992;21(3):315-17.

23. Zadikoff CM. Toxic encephalopathy associated with use of insect repellent. *J Pediatr* 1979;95:140-2.

24. Pronczuk de Garbino J and Laborda A. Toxicity of an insect repellent: N,N- diethyltoluamide. *Vet Hum Toxicol* 1983;25:422-3.

25. Hebert AA and Carlton S. Getting bugs to bug off: A review of insect repellents. *Contemp Pediatr* 1998;15:85-95.

26. Yolken R, Konecny P, and McCarthy P. Acute fluoride poisoning. *Pediatrics* 1976;58(1):90-3.

27. Heifetz SB and Horowitz HS. Amounts of fluoride in self-administered dental products: Safety considerations for children. *Pediatrics* 1986;77(6):876-82.

28. Gessner BD, Beler M, Middaugh JP, and Whitford GM. Acute fluoride poisoning from a public water system. *New Engl J Med* 1994;330(2):95-9.

29. Swanson L, Filandrinos DT, Shevlin JM, and Willett JR. Death from accidental ingestion of an ammonium and sodium bifluoride glass etching compound. *Vet Hum Toxicol* 1993;35(4):351.

30. Harchelroad F and Goetz C. Systemic fluoride intoxication with leukocytosis and pyrexia. *Vet Hum Toxicol* 1993;35(4):351.

31. Spak CJ, Sjöstedt S, Eleborg L, et al. Tissue response of gastric mucosa after ingestion of fluoride. *Br Med J* 1989;298:1686-7.

32. Baltazar RD, Mower MM, Reider R, et al. Acute fluoride poisoning leading to fatal hyperkalemia. *Chest* 1980;78:660.

33. Saunders LD, Ames RG, Knaak JB, et al. Outbreak of omite-cr-induced dermatitis among orange pickers in Tulare County, California. *J Occup Med* 1987;29:409-13.

34. Dorman DC and Beasley VR. Neurotoxicology of pyrethrin and the pyrethroid insecticides. *Vet Hum Toxicol* 1991;33(3):238-43.

35. He F, Wang S, Lui L, et al. Clinical manifestations and diagnosis of acute pyrethroid poisoning. *Arch Toxicol* 1989;63:54-8.

36. Tucker SB and Flannigan SA. Cutaneous effects from occupational exposure to fenvalerate. *Arch Toxicol* 1983;54:195-202.

37. Flannigan SA, Tucker SB, Key MM, et al. Synthetic pyrethroid insecticides: A dermatological evaluation. *Br J Ind Med* 1985;42:363-72.

38. Tucker SB, Flannigan SA, and Ross CE. Inhibitions of cutaneous paresthesia resulting from synthetic pyrethroid exposure. *Int J Dermatol* 1984;10:686-9.

39. O'Malley MA. Skin reactions to pesticides. *Occup Med* 1997;12:327-45.

40. Schwartz SM, Carroll HM, and Scharschmidt LA. Sublimed (inorganic) sulfur ingestion - A cause of life-threatening metabolic acidosis with a high anion gap. *Arch Intern Med* 1986;146:1437-8.

Section III

HERBICIDES

CHAPTER 9

Chlorophenoxy Herbicides

HIGHLIGHTS

Signs and Symptoms:

- Irritating to skin and mucous membranes

- Vomiting, diarrhea, headache, confusion, bizarre or aggressive behavior, peculiar odor on breath

- Metabolic acidosis, renal failure, tachycardia

Treatment:

- Washing, GI decontamination

- Administer IV

- Forced alkaline diuresis

Chlorophenoxy compounds are sometimes mixed into commercial fertilizers to control growth of broadleaf weeds. Several hundred commercial products contain chlorophenoxy herbicides in various forms, concentrations, and combinations. In some cases, the same name is used for products with different ingredients. The exact composition must therefore be determined from the product label. Sodium, potassium, and alkylamine salts are commonly formulated as aqueous solutions, while the less water-soluble esters are applied as emulsions. Low molecular weight esters are more volatile than the acids, salts, or long-chain esters.

Toxicology

Some of the chlorophenoxy acids, salts, and esters are moderately irritating to skin, eyes, and respiratory and gastrointestinal linings. In a few individuals, local depigmentation has apparently resulted from protracted dermal contact with chlorophenoxy compounds.

Chlorophenoxy compounds are well absorbed from the gastrointestinal tract.[1] They are less well absorbed from the lung. Cutaneous absorption appears to be minimal.[2] The compounds are not significantly stored in fat. Excretion occurs almost entirely by way of urine. Apart from some conjugation of the acids, there is limited biotransformation in the body.[1,2] The compounds are highly protein bound.[2] The average residence half-life of 2,4–D in humans is between 13 and 39 hours,[1,3,4,5] while that of 2,4,5–T is about 24 hours. Excretion is greatly enhanced in alkaline urine,[4,5,6] and with a half-life as prolonged as 70-90 hours with acidic urine.[6] Half-life is also longer with large doses and prolonged exposure.

Given in large doses to experimental animals, 2,4–D causes vomiting, diarrhea, anorexia, weight loss, ulcers of the mouth and pharynx, and toxic injury to the liver, kidneys, and central nervous system. Myotonia (stiffness and incoordination of hind extremities) develops in some species and is apparently due to CNS damage: demyelination has been observed in the dorsal columns of the cord, and EEG changes have indicated functional disturbances in the brains of heavily-dosed experimental animals.

Ingestion of large amounts of chlorophenoxy acids has resulted in severe metabolic acidosis in humans. Such cases have been associated with electrocardiographic changes, myotonia, muscle weakness, myoglobinuria, and elevated serum creatine phosphokinase, all reflecting injury to striated muscle. Chlorophenoxy acids are weak uncouplers of oxidative phosphorylation; therefore, extraordinary doses may produce hyperthermia from increased production of body heat.[5]

In the manufacture of some of these herbicides, other more toxic substances can be formed at excessive temperatures. These include chlorinated dibenzo dioxin (CDD) and chlorinated dibenzo furan (CDF). The 2,3,7,8-tetra CDD form is extraordinarily toxic to multiple mammalian tissues; it is formed only in the synthesis of 2,4,5-T. Hexa-, hepta-, and octa-compounds exhibit less systemic toxicity, but are the likely cause of chloracne (a chronic, disfiguring skin condition) seen in workers engaged in the manufacture of 2,4,5-T and certain other chlorinated organic compounds.[7] Although toxic effects, notably chloracne, have been observed in manufacturing plant workers, these effects have not been observed in formulators or applicators regularly exposed to 2,4,5-T or other chlorophenoxy compounds. All uses of 2,4,5-T in the U.S. have been cancelled.

The medical literature contains reports of peripheral neuropathy following what seemed to be minor dermal exposures to 2,4-D.[8] It is not certain that exposures to other neurotoxicants were entirely excluded in these cases. Single doses of 5 mg/kg body weight of 2,4-D and 2,4,5-T have been administered to human subjects without any adverse effects. One subject consumed 500 mg of 2,4-D per day for 3 weeks without experiencing symptoms or signs of illness.

Signs and Symptoms of Poisoning

Chlorophenoxy compounds are moderately irritating to skin and mucous membranes. Inhalation of sprays may cause burning sensations in the nasopharynx and chest, and coughing may result. Prolonged inhalation sometimes causes dizziness. Adjuvant chemicals added to enhance foliage penetration might account for the irritant effects of some formulations.

Manifestations of systemic toxicity of chlorophenoxy compounds are known mainly from clinical experience with cases of deliberate suicidal ingestion of large quantities. Most reports of fatal outcomes involve renal failure, acidosis, electrolyte imbalance, and a resultant multiple organ failure.[3,6,9] The agents most often involved in these incidents have been 2,4-D and mecoprop. The toxic effects of other chlorophenoxy compounds are probably similar but not identical.

Patients will present within a few hours of ingestion with vomiting, diarrhea, headache, confusion, and bizarre or aggressive behavior. Mental status changes occur with progression to coma in severe cases.[4,5,6] A peculiar odor is often noticed on the breath. Body temperature may be moderately elevated, but this is rarely a life-threatening feature of the poisoning. The respiratory drive is not depressed. Conversely, hyperventilation is sometimes evident, prob-

2,4-dichlorophenoxyacetic acid (2,4-D)
2,4-dichlorophenoxypropionic acid (2,4-DP)
  dichlorprop
2,4-dichlorophenoxybutyric acid (2,4-DB)
2,4,5-trichlorophenoxy acetic acid (2,4,5-T)
MCPA
MCPB
mecoprop (MCPP)
2-methyl-3, 6 dichlorobenzoic acid
  Banvel
  Dicamba

ably secondary to the metabolic acidosis that occurs. Muscle weakness and peripheral neuropathy have been reported after occupational exposure.[6] Convulsions occur very rarely. With effective urinary excretion of the toxicant, consciousness usually returns in 48-96 hours.[4,5,6]

As mentioned above, chlorophenoxy compounds cause significant metabolic changes. Metabolic acidosis is manifest as a low arterial pH and bicarbonate content. The urine is usually acidic. Skeletal muscle injury, if it occurs, is reflected in elevated creatine phosphokinase, and sometimes myoglobinuria. Moderate elevations of blood urea nitrogen and serum creatinine are commonly found as the toxicant is excreted. Cases of renal failure are reported, often with an accompanying hyperkalemia or hypocalcemia that was thought to result in the cardiovascular instability that led to death.[3,9] Tachycardia is commonly observed, and hypotension has also been reported.[3,4,6] T-wave flattening has also been observed.[5] Mild leukocytosis and biochemical changes indicative of liver cell injury have been reported.

Myotonia and muscle weakness may persist for months after acute poisoning.[5] Electromyographic and nerve conduction studies in some recovering patients have demonstrated a mild proximal neuropathy and myopathy.

Confirmation of Poisoning

Gas-liquid chromatographic methods are available for detecting chlorophenoxy compounds in blood and urine. These analyses are useful in confirming and assessing the magnitude of chlorophenoxy absorption. Poisoning characterized by unconsciousness has shown initial blood chlorophenoxy concentrations ranging from 80 to more than 1000 mg per liter.[4] Urine samples should be collected as soon as possible after exposure because the herbicides may be almost completely excreted in 24-72 hours under normal conditions. Urine samples can also confirm overexposure. In a study of asymptomatic herbicide applicators, their urinary excretion of chlorophenoxy compounds rarely exceeded 1-2 mg/L.[10] The half-life may be much longer in cases of intoxication depending on the extent of absorption and urine pH.

Analyses can be performed at special laboratories usually known to local poison control centers. If the clinical scenario indicates that excessive exposure to chlorophenoxy compounds has occurred, initiate appropriate treatment measures immediately. Do not wait for chemical confirmation of toxicant absorption.

Treatment

1. Precautions. Individuals with chronic skin disease or known sensitivity to these herbicides should either avoid using them or take strict precautions to avoid contact (respirator, gloves, etc.).

2. Respiratory protection. If any symptoms of illness occur during or following inhalation of spray, remove victim from contact with the material for at least 2-3 days. Allow subsequent contact with chlorophenoxy compounds only if effective respiratory protection is practiced.

3. Skin decontamination. Flush contaminating chemicals from eyes with copious amounts of clean water for 10-15 minutes. If irritation persists, an ophthalmologic examination should be performed.

4. Gastrointestinal decontamination. If substantial amounts of chlorophenoxy compounds have been ingested, spontaneous emesis may occur. Gastric decontamination procedures may be considered, as outlined in Chapter 2.

5. Intravenous fluids. Administer intravenous fluids to accelerate excretion of the chlorophenoxy compound, and to limit concentration of the toxicant in the kidney. A urine flow of 4-6 mL/minute is desirable. Intravenous saline/dextrose has sufficed to rescue comatose patients who drank 2,4-D and mecoprop several hours before hospital admission.

    Caution: Monitor urine protein and cells, BUN, serum creatinine, serum electrolytes, and fluid intake/output carefully to insure that renal function remains unimpaired and that fluid overload does not occur.

6. Diuresis. Forced alkaline diuresis has been used successfully in management of suicidal ingestions of chlorophenoxy compounds, especially when initiated early.[4,5,6] Alkalinizing the urine by including sodium bicarbonate (44-88 mEq per liter) in the intravenous solution accelerates excretion of 2,4-D dramatically and mecoprop excretion substantially. Urine pH should be maintained between 7.6 and 8.8. Include potassium chloride as needed to offset increased potassium losses: add 20-40 mEq of potassium chloride to each liter of intravenous solution. It is crucial to monitor serum electrolytes carefully, especially potassium and calcium.

    There may possibly be some hazard to the kidneys when urine concentrations of toxicant are very high, so the integrity of renal function and fluid balance should be monitored carefully as the chlorophenoxy compound is excreted. Renal failure has occurred in patients with severe intoxication during alkaline diuresis. In one case, the diuresis was begun 26 hours after ingestion,[6] and the other two were initiated a couple days after poisoning.[3,9]

7. Hemodialysis is not likely to be of significant benefit in poisonings by chlorophenoxy compounds. It has been used in four patients who survived intoxication.[11] However, given the highly protein-bound nature of these herbicides and lack of any other evidence, hemodialysis is not recommended.[2]

8. Follow-up clinical examination should include electromyographic and nerve conduction studies to detect any neuropathic changes and neuromuscular junction defects.

General Chemical Structure

References

1. Kohli JD, Khanna RN, Gupta BN, et al. Absorption and excretion of 2,4-dichlorophenoxyacetic. *Xenobiotica* 1974;4(2):97-100.

2. Arnold EK, Beasley MS, and Beasley VR. The pharmacokinetics of chlorinated phenoxy acid Herbicides: A literature review. *Vet Hum Toxicol* 1989;31(2):121-5.

3. Keller T, Skopp G, Wu M, et al. Fatal overdose of 2,4-dichlorophenoxyacetic acid (2,4-D). *Forensic Sci Int* 1994;65:13-8.

4. Friesen EG, Jones GR, and Vaughan D. Clinical presentation and management of acute 2,4-D oral ingestion. *Drug Saf* 1990;5(2):155-90.

5. Prescott LF, Park J, and Darrien I. Treatment of severe 2,4-D and mecoprop intoxication with alkaline diuresis. *Bri Journal of Clinical Pharmacology* 1979;7:111-116.

6. Flanagan RJ, Meredith TJ, Ruprah M, et al. Alkaline diuresis for acute poisoning with chlorophenoxy herbicides and ioxynil. *Lancet* 1990;335:454-8.

7. Poskitt LB, Duffill MB, and Rademaker M. Chloracne, palmoplantar keratoderma and localized scleroderma in a weed sprayer. *Clin and Exp Dermatol* 1994; 19:264-7.

8. O'Reilly JF. Prolonged coma and delayed peripheral neuropathy after ingestion of phenoxyacetic acid weedkillers. *Postgrad Med Journal* 1984;60:76-7.

9. Kancir CB, Anderson C, and Olesen AS. Marked hypocalcemia in a fatal poisoning with chlorinated phenoxy acid derivatives. *Clin Toxicol* 26(3&4):257-64.

10. Kolmodin-Hedman B, Hoglund S, and Akerblom M. Studies on phenoxy acid herbicides, I, Field study: Occupational exposure to phenoxy acid herbicides (MCPA, dichlorprop, mecoprop, and 2,4-D) in agriculture. *Arch Toxicol* 1983;54:257-65.

11. Durakovic Z, Durakovic A, Durakovic S, et al. Poisoning with 2,4- dichlorophenoxyacetic acid treated by hemodialysis. *Arch Toxicol* 1992;66:518-21.

CHAPTER 10

Pentachlorophenol

HIGHLIGHTS

- Absorbed by skin, lung, GI lining
- Fatalities reported, associated with intensive exposure in hot environments

Signs and Symptoms:

- Irritation of the nose, throat, and eyes
- Hyperthermia, muscle spasm, tremor, labored breathing, and chest tightness indicate serious poisoning

Treatment:

- No specific antidote
- Control fever, replace fluids, oxygen
- Decontaminate eyes, skin, hair, clothing
- Monitor cardiac status, control agitation

Contraindicated:

- Salicylates for fever control

Pentachlorophenol (PCP) is currently registered in the United States only as a restricted use pesticide for use as a wood preservative. PCP has been used as an herbicide, algacide, defoliant, wood preservative, germicide, fungicide, and molluscicide.[1] As a wood preservative, it is commonly applied as a 0.1% solution in mineral spirits, No. 2 fuel oil, or kerosene. It is used in pressure treatment of lumber at 5% concentration. Weed killers have contained higher concentrations.

Pentachlorophenol volatilizes from treated wood and fabric. It has a significant phenolic odor, which becomes quite strong when the material is heated. Excessively treated interior surfaces may be a source of exposure sufficient to cause irritation of eyes, nose, and throat.

Technical PCP contains lower chlorinated phenols (4–12%) plus traces of chlorobenzodioxins, chlorobenzofurans, and chlorobenzenes. Incomplete combustion of PCP-treated wood may lead to the formation of these compounds.

Toxicology

PCP is readily absorbed across the skin, the lungs, and the gastrointestinal lining. In animals, the dermal LD_{50} is of the same order of magnitude as the oral. With acute exposure it is rapidly excreted, mainly in the urine, as unchanged PCP and as PCP glucuronide. In chronic exposures, the elimination half-life has been reported to be very long, up to 20 days.[2] In another study, three volunteers took consecutive oral doses of PCP, and a half-life of 20 days was also found. The long half-life was attributed to the low urinary clearance because of high protein binding.[3] In the blood, a large fraction of absorbed PCP is protein-bound. It is widely distributed to other tissues in the body, including kidney, heart, and adrenal glands.

At certain concentrations, PCP is irritating to mucous membranes and skin. Contact dermatitis is common among workers having contact with PCP. In a study of employees involved in the manufacture of PCP, chloracne was found in 7% of the workers, and the risk was significantly higher among employees with documented skin contact compared to employees without skin contact.[4] Urticaria has also been reported as an uncommon response in exposed persons.

The primary toxicological mechanism is increased cellular oxidative metabolism resulting from the uncoupling of oxidative phosphorylation. Heat production is increased and leads to clinical hyperthermia. This clinical state may mimic the signs and symptoms found in hyperthyroidism. Internally, large doses are toxic to the liver, kidneys, and nervous system.

Based on laboratory experimentation on animals, PCP has been reported to have fetotoxic and embrotoxic properties and to bind to various hormone receptors.[5,6] Epidemiological evidence suggests exposed persons may be at risk for miscarriages, reduced birth weight, and other malformations.[7,8]

Albuminuria, glycosuria, aminoaciduria, and elevated BUN reflect renal injury. Liver enlargement, anemia, and leukopenia have been reported in some intensively exposed workers. Elevated serum alkaline phosphatase, AST, and LDH enzymes indicate significant insult to the liver, including both cellular damage and some degree of biliary obstruction.

Signs and Symptoms of Poisoning

The most common effects of airborne PCP include local irritation of the nose, throat, and eyes, producing a stuffy nose, scratchy throat, and tearing. Dermal exposure is also common and may lead to irritation, contact dermatitis, or more rarely, diffuse urticaria or chloracne. Individual cases of exfoliative dermatitis of the hands and diffuse urticaria and angioedema of the hands have been reported in intensively exposed workers. Several infant deaths occurred in a nursery where a PCP-containing diaper rinse had been used.

Severe poisoning and death have occurred as a result of intensive PCP exposure. Acute poisoning occurs with systemic absorption which can occur by any route of sufficient dosage. Most occupational poisonings occur through dermal contact. Hyperthermia, muscle spasm, tremor, labored breathing, and chest tightness indicate serious poisoning. The patient may also complain of abdominal pain, and exhibit vomiting, restlessness, and mental confusion. Tachycardia and increased respiratory rate are usually apparent. Other commonly reported signs and symptoms of systemic poisoning include profuse sweating, weakness, dizziness, anorexia, and intense thirst. Workers exposed over long periods may experience weight loss.

Most adult fatalities have occurred in persons working in hot environments where hyperthermia is poorly tolerated. Cases of aplastic anemia and leukemia have been reported which were associated temporally with PCP exposure. Causal relationships in these cases were not established.[9] Peripheral neuropathies have also been reported in some cases of long-term occupational exposure; however, a causal relationship has not been supported by longitudinal studies.[10]

Confirmation of Poisoning

If poisoning is strongly suspected on the basis of exposure, symptoms, and signs, **do not postpone treatment** until diagnosis is confirmed.

PCP can be measured in blood, urine, and adipose tissue by gas-liquid chromatography. Plasma levels can be much greater than urine levels (ratio of blood to urine is 1.0 to 2.5) so care must be taken in interpreting results.[10,11] There is no clear-cut determination of what constitutes an abnormally high level of PCP, and there is great variability among different references. Most information on the extent of serum levels in relation to toxicity is based on individual cases or small series of patients. Reports exist of asymptomatic infants with serum levels as high as 26 parts per million (ppm).[11,12] However, most reports of non–occupational exposure in the general public involve levels in the parts per billion range.[1,13-15] Food is probably the main source of this nanogram-level dosage.[1] Serum levels among occupationally exposed persons often exceed 1 ppm.[1] A report of a lethal case describes a plasma level of 16 ppm,[16] but most cases generally involve serum levels in the range of 100 ppm or higher.[11,17] It is reasonable to assume that levels greater than 1 ppm are consistent with an unusual exposure and that levels approaching 100 ppm are cause for great concern.

Treatment

1. Supportive treatment and hyperthermia control. There is no specific antidote to the poisoning; therefore treatment is supportive in nature including oxygen, fluid replacement, and most importantly, fever control.

Reduce elevated body temperature by physical means. Administer sponge baths and use fans to increase evaporation.[18] In fully conscious patients, administer cold, sugar-containing liquids by mouth as tolerated. Cooling blankets and ice packs to body surfaces may also be used.

Antipyretic therapy with salicylates is **strongly contraindicated** as salicylates also uncouple oxidative phosphorylation. Other antipyretics are thought to be of no use because of the peripherally mediated mechanism of hyperthermia in poisoning of this nature. Neither the safety nor the effectiveness of the other antipyretics has been tested.

Administer oxygen continuously by mask to minimize tissue anoxia. Unless there are manifestations of cerebral or pulmonary edema or of inadequate renal function, administer intravenous fluids to restore hydration and support physiologic mechanisms for heat loss and toxicant disposition. Monitor serum electrolytes, adjusting IV infusions to stabilize electrolyte concentrations. Follow urine contents of albumin and cells, and keep an accurate hourly record of intake/output to forestall fluid overload if renal function declines.

Caution: In the presence of cerebral edema and/or impaired renal function, intravenous fluids must be administered very cautiously to avoid increased intracranial pressure and pulmonary edema. Central monitoring of venous and pulmonary wedge pressures may be indicated. Such critically ill patients should be treated in an intensive care unit.

2. Skin decontamination. Flush the chemical from eyes with copious amounts of clean water. Perform skin decontamination as described in Chapter 2.

3. Cardiopulmonary monitoring. In severe poisonings, monitor pulmonary status carefully to insure adequate gas exchange, and monitor cardiac status by ECG to detect arrhythmias. The toxicant itself and severe electrolyte disturbances may predispose to arrhythmias and myocardial weakness.

4. Neurological. To reduce production of heat in the body, control agitation and involuntary motor activity with sedation. Lorazepam or other benzodiazepines should be effective, although use of these drugs in these poisonings has not been reported. If lorazepam is chosen, administer slowly, intravenously.

Dosage of Lorazepam:

- *Adults:* 2-4 mg/dose IV given over 2-5 minutes. Repeat if necessary to a maximum of 8 mg in a 12-hour period.

- *Adolescents:* Same as adult dose, except maximum dose is 4 mg.

- *Children under 12 years:* 0.05-0.10 mg/kg IV over 2-5 minutes. Repeat if necessary 0.05 mg/kg 10-15 minutes after first dose, with a maximum dose of 4 mg.

Caution: Be prepared to assist pulmonary ventilation mechanically if respiration is depressed, to intubate the trachea if laryngospasm occurs, and to counteract hypotensive reactions.

---

5. Gastrointestinal decontamination. If PCP has been ingested in a quantity sufficient to cause poisoning and the patient presents within one hour, consider gastric decontamination as outlined in Chapter 2.

6. Nutrition. During convalescence, administer a high-calorie, high-vitamin diet to restore body fat and carbohydrates. Discourage subsequent contact with the toxicant for 4-8 weeks (depending on severity of poisoning) to allow full restoration of normal metabolic processes.

Chemical Structure

References

1. Jorens PG and Schepens PJC. Human pentachlorophenol poisoning. *Hum Exp Toxicol* 1993;479-95.

2. Kalman DA and Horstman SW. Persistence of tetrachlorophenol and pentachlorophenol in exposed woodworkers. *J Toxicol Clin Toxicol* 1983;20:343.

3. Uhl S, Schmid P, and Schlatter C. Pharmacokinetics of pentachlorophenol in man. *Arch Toxicol* 1986;58:182-6.

4. O'Malley MA, Carpenter AV, Sweeney MH, et al. Chloracne associated with employment in the production of pentachlorophenol. *Am J Ind Med* 1990;17:411-21.

5. Danzo BJ. Environmental xenobiotics may disrupt normal endocrine function by interfering with the binding of physiological ligands to steroid receptors and binding proteins. *Environ Health Perspect* 1997;105:294-301.

6. Tran DQ, Klotz DM, Ladlie BL, et al. Inhibition of progesterone receptor activity in yeast by synthetic chemicals. *Biochem Biophys Res Commun* 1996;229:518-23.

7. Dimich-Ward H, Hertzman C, Teschke K, et al. Reproductive effects of paternal exposure to chlorophenate wood preservatives in the sawmill industry. *Scand J Work Environ Health* 1996;22:267-73.

8. DeMaeyer J, Schepens PJ, Jorens PG, and Verstaete R. Exposure to pentachlorophenol as a possible cause of miscarriages. *Br J Obstet Gynaecol* 1995;102:1010-1.

9. Roberts HJ. Aplastic anemia due to pentachlorophenol. *New Engl J Med* 1981;305:1650-1.

10. Casarett LJ, Bevenue A, Yauger WL, and Whalen SA. Observations on pentachlorophenol in human blood and urine. *Am Ind Hyg Assoc J* 1969;30:360-6.

11. Clayton GD and Clayton FE (eds). Patty's Industrial Hygiene and Toxicology, vol 2B, 4th ed. New York: John Wiley & Sons, 1994, pp. 1605-13.

12. Robson AM, Kissane JM, Elvick WH, et al. Pentachlorophenol poisoning in a nursery for newborn infants: Clinical features and treatment. *J Pediatr* 1969;75:309-16.

13. Gomez-Catalan J, To-Figueras J, Planas J, et al. Pentachlorophenol and hexachlorobenzene in serum and urine of the population of Barcelona. *Hum Toxicol* 1987;6:397-400.

14. Wylie JA, Gabica J, Benson WW, and Yoder J. Exposure and contamination of the air and employees of a pentachlorophenol plant, Idaho-1972. *Pest Monit J* 1975;9:150-3.

15. Wagner SL. Pentachlorophenol. In: Clinical Toxicology of Agricultural Chemicals. Corvallis, OR: Oregon State University Press, 1981, pp. 131-7.

16. Wood S, Rom WN, White GL, and Logan DC. Pentachlorophenol poisoning. *J Occup Med* 1983;25:527-30.

17. Gray RE, Gilliland RD, Smith EE, et al. Pentachlorophenol intoxication: Report of a fatal case, with comments on the clinical course and pathologic anatomy. *Arch Environ Health* 1985;40:161-4.

18. Graham BS, Lichtenstein MJ, Hinson JM, et al. Nonexertional heatstroke: Physiologic management and cooling in 14 patients. *Arch Intern Med* 1986;146:87-90.

Nitrophenolic and Nitrocresolic Herbicides

These highly toxic chemicals have many uses in agriculture worldwide, as herbicides (weed-killing and defoliation), acaricides, nematocides, ovicides, and fungicides. Relatively insoluble in water, most technical products are dissolved in organic solvents and formulated for spray application as emulsions. There are some wettable powder formulations. Only dinocap continues to have active registrations in the United States.

Toxicology

Nitroaromatic compounds are highly toxic to humans and animals with LD_{50}s in the range of 25 to 50 mg/kg.[1] Most nitrophenols and nitrocresols are well absorbed by the skin, gastrointestinal tract, or lung when fine droplets are inhaled.[2] Fatal poisonings have occurred as a result of dermal contamination; more common is a moderate irritation of the skin and mucous membranes.

Nitrophenols and nitrocresols undergo some biotransformation in humans, chiefly reduction (one nitro group to an amino group) and conjugation at the phenolic site. Although nitrophenols and metabolites appear consistently in the urine of poisoned individuals, hepatic excretion is probably the main route of disposition. Elimination is slow with a documented half-life in humans between 5 and 14 days.[1] Blood and tissue concentrations tend to increase progressively if an individual is substantially exposed on successive days.

The basic mechanism of toxicity is stimulation of oxidative metabolism in cell mitochondria, by the uncoupling of oxidative phosphorylation. This leads to hyperthermia, tachycardia, headache, malaise, and dehydration, and in time, depletes carbohydrate and fat stores. The major systems prone to toxicity are the hepatic, renal, and nervous systems. The nitrophenols are more active as uncouplers than chlorophenols such as pentachlorophenol (described in chapter 10). Hyperthermia and direct toxicity on the brain cause restlessness and headache, and in severe cases, seizures, coma, and cerebral edema. The higher the ambient temperature, such as in an outdoor agricultural environment, the more difficult it is to dissipate the heat.[1,2] Liver parenchyma and renal tubules show degenerative changes. Albuminuria, pyuria, hematuria, and azotemia are signs of renal injury.

Cataracts occur in laboratory animals given nitrophenols, and have occurred in humans, both as a result of ill-advised medicinal use and as a consequence of chronic, occupational exposure.[3] Cataract formation is sometimes accompanied by glaucoma.

Signs and Symptoms of Poisoning

Most patients present within a few hours of exposure with generalized non-specific signs and symptoms including profuse sweating, thirst, fever, headache, confusion, malaise, and restlessness. The skin may appear warm and flushed as **hyperthermia** develops, along with tachycardia, and tachypnea, all of which indicate a serious degree of poisoning. Apprehension, anxiety, manic behavior, seizures, and coma reflect cerebral injury; seizures and coma signify an immediately life-threatening intoxication. Labored breathing and cyanosis are consequences of the stimulated metabolism and tissue anoxia. Renal failure may occur early in cases of severe exposure. Liver damage is first manifested by jaundice, and cell death can occur within 48 hours and is dose-dependent.[4] Death may occur within 24 to 48 hours after exposure in cases of severe poisoning.[2] In cases of survival of severe poisoning, complete resolution of symptoms may be slow due to the toxicant's long half-life.[1,5]

A characteristic bright yellow staining of skin and hair is often present with topical exposure and can be an important diagnostic clue to the clinician.[1,2,5] Yellow staining of the sclerae and urine indicates absorption of potentially toxic amounts. Weight loss occurs in persons continually exposed to relatively low doses of nitrophenols or nitrocresols.[1,3]

Confirmation of Poisoning

If poisoning is probable, do not await confirmation before beginning treatment. Save urine and blood specimens on ice at temperature below 20° C in the event confirmation is necessary later on. Unmetabolized nitrophenols and nitrocresols can be identified spectrophotometrically, or by gas-liquid chromatography, in the serum at concentrations well below those that have been associated with acute poisonings. The data on exposure and systemic levels of compounds in this group are limited, and most reports specify the compound dinitro-ortho-cresol. In general, blood levels of 10 mcg/dL or greater are usually seen when systemic toxicity is evident.[1,6] One fatal case occured with a level of 75 mcg/dL.[6] Blood analysis is useful in confirming the cause of poisoning. Monitoring of levels should be done routinely during acute intoxication in order to establish a decay curve to determine when therapy can be safely discontinued.

Treatment

1. Supportive treatment and hyperthermia control. There is no specific antidote to poisoning with nitrophenolic or nitrocresolic herbicides. Treatment is supportive in nature and includes oxygen, fluid replacement, and temperature control.

Reduce elevated body temperature by physical means. Administer sponge baths and ice packs, and use a fan to promote air flow and evaporation.[7] In fully conscious patients, administer cold, sugar-containing liquids by mouth as tolerated.

2. Contraindications. Antipyretic therapy with salicylates is strongly contraindicated as salicylates also uncouple oxidative phosphorylation. Other antipyretics are thought to be of no use because of the peripherally mediated mechanism of hyperthermia in poisoning of this nature. Neither the safety nor the effectiveness of other antipyretics has been tested.

Atropine is also absolutely contraindicated! It is essential not to confuse the clinical signs for dinitrophenol with manifestations for cholinesterase inhibition poisoning.[2]

3. Skin decontamination. If poisoning has been caused by contamination of body surfaces, bathe and shampoo contaminated skin and hair promptly and thoroughly with soap and water, or water alone if soap is not available. Wash the chemical from skin folds and from under fingernails. Care should be taken to prevent dermal contamination of hospital staff. See Chapter 2.

4. Other Treatment. Other aspects of treatment are identical to management of pentachlorophenol poisoning, detailed in Chapter 10.

General Chemical Structure

References

1. Leftwich RB, Floro JF, Neal RA, et al. Dinitrophenol poisoning: A diagnosis to consider in undiagnosed fever. *South Med J* 1982;75:182-5.

2. Finkel AJ. Herbicides: Dinitrophenols. In: Hamilton and Hardy's Industrial Toxicology, 4th ed. Boston: John Wright PSG, Inc., 1983, pp. 301-2.

3. Kurt TL, Anderson R, Petty C, et al. Dinitrophenol in weight loss: The poison center and public safety. *Vet Hum Toxicol* 1986;28:574-5.

4. Palmeira CM, Moreno AJ, and Madeira VM. Thiols metabolism is altered by the herbicides paraquat, dinoseb, and 2.4-D: A study in isolated hepatocytes. *Toxicol Lett* 1995;81:115-23.

5. Smith WD. An investigation of suspected dinoseb poisoning after agricultural use of a herbicide. *Practitioner* 1981;225:923-6.

6. NIOSH. Criteria document: Occupational exposure to dinitro-orthocresol. Cincinnati: NIOSH, 1978.

7. Graham BS, Lichtenstein MJ, Hinson JM, et al. Nonexertional heatstroke: Physiologic management and cooling in 14 patients. *Arch Intern Med* 1986;146:87-90.

Paraquat and Diquat

HIGHLIGHTS

- Life-threatening effects on GI tract, kidney, liver, heart, other organs
- Pulmonary fibrosis is the usual cause of death in paraquat poisoning (but not diquat)

Signs and Symptoms:

- Paraquat and diquat (ingestion): burning pain in the mouth, throat, chest, upper abdomen; pulmonary edema, pancreatitis, other renal, CNS effects
- Paraquat (dermal): dry and fissured hands, horizontal ridging or loss of fingernails, ulceration and abrasion
- Diquat: neurologic toxicity

Treatment:

- Immediate GI decontamination with Bentonite, Fuller's Earth, or activated charcoal
- Maintain urinary output by administering IV, but monitor fluids in case of renal failure
- Decontaminate eyes and skin

Contraindicated:

- No supplemental oxygen unless patient develops severe hypoxemia

The dipyridyl compounds paraquat and diquat are non-selective contact herbicides that are relatively widely-used, primarily in agriculture and by government agencies and industries for control of weeds. While paraquat is a restricted-use pesticide in most forms for most uses in the United States, its wide usage leads to significant potential for misuse and accidental and intentional poisonings. In the past few decades, paraquat has been a popular agent for suicide, but recent experience indicates a decline in such intentional poisonings. Paraquat and diquat are highly toxic compounds and management of poisonings requires a great deal of skill and knowledge of proper management procedures.

PARAQUAT

Toxicology

When ingested in adequate dosage (see below), paraquat has life-threatening effects on the gastrointestinal tract, kidney, liver, heart, and other organs. The LD_{50} in humans is approximately 3–5 mg/kg, which translates into as little as 10–15 mL of a 20% solution.[1,2]

The lung is the primary target organ of paraquat, and pulmonary effects represent the most lethal and least treatable manifestation of toxicity. However, toxicity from inhalation is rare. The primary mechanism is through the generation of free radicals with oxidative damage to lung tissue.[1,2] While acute pulmonary edema and early lung damage may occur within a few hours of severe acute exposures,[3,4] the delayed toxic damage of pulmonary fibrosis, the usual cause of death, most commonly occurs 7–14 days after the ingestion.[5] In patients who ingested a very large amount of concentrated solution (20%), some have died more rapidly (within 48 hours) from circulatory failure.[5]

Both types I and II pneumatocytes appear to selectively accumulate paraquat. Biotransformation of paraquat in these cells results in free-radical production with resulting lipid peroxidation and cell injury.[1,2,4] Hemorrhage proteinaceous edema fluid and leukocytes infiltrate the alveolar spaces, after which there is rapid proliferation of fibroblasts. There is a progressive decline in arterial oxygen tension and CO_2 diffusion capacity. Such a severe impairment of gas exchange causes progressive proliferation of fibrous connective tissue in the alveoli and eventual death from asphyxia and tissue anoxia.[6] One prospective study of survivors suggests that some of the fibrous toxic damage may be reversible as evidence exists of markedly improved pulmonary function three months after survival.[7]

Local skin damage includes contact dermatitis. Prolonged contact will produce erythema, blistering, abrasion and ulceration, and fingernail changes.[8,9] Although absorption across intact skin is slow, abraded or eroded skin allows efficient absorption.

The gastrointestinal (GI) tract is the site of initial or phase I toxicity to the mucosal surfaces following ingestion of the substance. This toxicity is manifested by swelling, edema, and painful ulceration of the mouth, pharynx, esophagus, stomach, and intestine. With higher levels, other GI toxicity includes centrizonal hepatocellular injury which can cause elevated bilirubin, and hepatocellular enzymes such as AST, ALT, and LDH.

Damage to the proximal renal tubule is often more reversible than the destruction to lung tissue. However, impaired renal function may play a critical role in determining the outcome of paraquat poisoning. Normal tubule cells actively secrete paraquat into the urine, efficiently clearing it from the blood. However, high blood concentrations poison the secretory mechanism and may destroy the cells. Diquat poisoning typically results in greater renal injury compared to paraquat.

Focal necrosis of the myocardium and skeletal muscle are the main features of toxicity to any type of muscle tissue, and typically occur as a second phase. Ingestion has also been reported to cause cerebral edema and brain damage.[10]

Although much concern has been expressed about the effects of smoking paraquat-contaminated marijuana, toxic effects caused by this mechanism have been either very rare or nonexistent. Most paraquat that contaminates marijuana is pyrolyzed during smoking to dipyridyl, which is a product of combustion of the leaf material itself (including marijuana) and presents little toxic hazard.

Signs and Symptoms of Poisoning

Initial clinical signs depend upon the route of exposure. Early symptoms and signs of poisoning by ingestion are burning pain in the mouth, throat, chest, and upper abdomen, due to the corrosive effect of paraquat on the mucosal lining. Diarrhea, which is sometimes bloody, can also occur. Giddiness, headache, fever, myalgia, lethargy, and coma are other examples of CNS and systemic findings. Pancreatitis may cause severe abdominal pain. Proteinuria, hematuria, pyuria, and azotemia reflect renal injury. Oliguria/anuria indicate acute tubular necrosis.

Because the kidney is almost the exclusive route of paraquat elimination from body tissues, renal failure fosters a build-up of tissue concentrations, including those in the lung. Unfortunately, this pathogenic sequence may occur in the first several hours following paraquat ingestion, generating lethal concentrations of paraquat in lung tissue before therapeutic measures to limit absorption and enhance disposition have taken effect. It is probably for this reason

Commercial Products

PARAQUAT

Liquid Concentrates:
Cekuquat
Crisquat
Dextrone
Esgram
Goldquat
Gramocil
Gramonol
Gramoxone

In combination with other herbicides:
With diquat:
　Actor
　Preeglone
　Preglone
　Weedol (a 2.5% soluble
　granule formulation)

With diuron:
　Dexuron
　Gramuron
　Para-col
　Tota-col

With monolinuron:
　Gramonol

With simazine:
　Pathclear
　Terraklene

DIQUAT

Aquacide
Dextrone
Ortho Diquat
Reglone

that methods for enhancing paraquat disposition several hours following ingestion have had little effect on mortality.

Cough, dyspnea, and tachypnea usually appear 2–4 days following paraquat ingestion, but may be delayed as long as 14 days. Progressive cyanosis and dyspnea reflect deteriorating gas exchange in the damaged lung. In some cases, the coughing up of frothy sputum (pulmonary edema) is the early and principal manifestation of paraquat lung injury.

Clinical experience has offered a rough dose–effect scale on which to base prognosis in cases of paraquat ingestion:[9]

- **Less than 20 mg** paraquat ion per kg body weight (less than 7.5 mL of 20% [w/v] paraquat concentrate): No symptoms or only gastrointestinal symptoms occur. Recovery is likely.

- **Twenty to 40 mg** paraquat ion per kg body weight (7.5–15.0 mL of 20% [w/v] paraquat concentrate): Pulmonary fibroplasia ensues. Death occurs in most cases, but may be delayed 2–3 weeks.

- **More than 40 mg** paraquat ion per kg body weight (more than 15.0 mL of 20% [w/v] paraquat concentrate): Multiple organ damage occurs as in class II, but is more rapidly progressive. Often characterized by marked ulceration of the oropharynx. Mortality is essentially 100% in 1–7 days.

Dermal signs are common among agriculture workers with acute paraquat toxicity. Particularly in concentrated form, paraquat causes localized injury to tissues with which it comes into contact. Fatal poisonings are reported to have occurred as a result of protracted dermal contamination by paraquat, but this is likely to occur only when the skin is abraded, eroded, or diseased, when more efficient systemic absorption can occur. With an intact dermal barrier, paraquat leaves the skin of the hands dry and fissured, can cause horizontal ridging of the fingernails, and may even result in the loss of fingernails. Prolonged contact with skin will create ulceration and abrasion, sufficient to allow systemic absorption.

In addition, some agriculture workers can be exposed through prolonged inhalation of spray droplets, and develop nosebleeds due to local damage. However, inhalation has not resulted in systemic toxicity, due to the low vapor pressure and lower concentration of paraquat field formulations. Eye contamination with diquat concentrate or stronger solutions results in severe conjunctivitis and sometimes protracted corneal opacification.

The hepatic injury from paraquat may be severe enough to cause jaundice, which signifies severe injury. However, hepatotoxicity is rarely a major determinant to clinical outcome. No other hepatic signs or symptoms are present other than the abnormal laboratory values mentioned in the Toxicology section.

DIQUAT

Toxicology

Diquat poisoning is much less common than paraquat poisoning, so that human reports and animal experimental data for diquat poisoning are less extensive than for paraquat. Systemically absorbed diquat is not selectively concentrated in lung tissue, as is paraquat, and pulmonary injury by diquat is less prominent. In animal studies, diquat causes mild, reversible injury to type I pneumatocytes, but does not injure the type II cells. No progressive pulmonary fibrosis has been noted in diquat poisoning.[11-13]

However, diquat has severe toxic effects on the central nervous system that are not typical of paraquat poisoning.[12,13] While laboratory experimentation has suggested that diquat is not directly neurotoxic, there have been relatively consistent pathologic brain changes noted in reported fatal cases of diquat poisoning. These consist of brain stem infarction, particularly involving the pons.[12] It is not clear whether these post-mortem changes represent direct toxicity or secondary effects related to the systemic illness and therapy. (See Signs and Symptoms section for CNS clinical effects.)

There is probably significant absorption of diquat across abraded or ulcerated skin.

Signs and Symptoms of Poisoning

In many human diquat poisoning cases, clinical signs of neurologic toxicity are the most important. These include nervousness, irritability, restlessness, combativeness, disorientation, nonsensical statements, inability to recognize friends or family members, and diminished reflexes. Neurologic effects may progress to coma, accompanied by tonic-clonic seizures, and result in the death of the patient.[12,13] Parkinsonism has also been reported following dermal exposure to diquat.[14]

Except for the CNS signs listed in the preceding paragraph, early symptoms of poisoning by ingested diquat are similar to those from paraquat, reflecting its corrosive effect on tissues. They include burning pain in the mouth, throat, chest, and abdomen, intense nausea and vomiting, and diarrhea. If the dosage was small, these symptoms may be delayed 1–2 days. Blood may appear in the vomitus and feces. Intestinal ileus, with pooling of fluid in the gut, has characterized several human poisonings by diquat.

The kidney is the principal excretory pathway for diquat absorbed into the body. Renal damage is therefore an important feature of poisonings. Proteinuria, hematuria, and pyuria may progress to renal failure and azotemia. Elevations of serum alkaline phosphatase, AST, ALT, and LDH reflect liver injury. Jaundice may develop.

If the patient survives several hours or days, circulatory function may fail due to dehydration. Hypotension and tachycardia can occur, with shock resulting in death. Other cardiorespiratory problems may develop, such as toxic cardiomyopathy or a secondary infection such as bronchopneumonia.

Diquat is somewhat less damaging to the skin than paraquat, but irritant effects may appear following dermal contamination with the concentrate. There is probably significant absorption of diquat across abraded or ulcerated skin.

The great majority of poisonings by paraquat and diquat (discussed below) have been caused by ingestion with suicidal intent in most cases, particularly in Japan[11] and many developing countries. Since 1987, there has been a decline in most countries in the total numbers of suicidal deaths attributed to paraquat and diquat. Nearly all of the few poisonings caused by occupational exposure have been survived, but the mortality rate among persons who have swallowed paraquat or diquat remains high.[1,5] Avoidance of this mortality will probably have to rely on preventive strategies or on stopping gastrointestinal absorption very soon after the toxicant has been ingested.

Even though intestinal absorption of dipyridyls is relatively slow, lethal uptake by critical organs and tissues apparently occurs within 18 hours, and possibly within 6 hours, following ingestion of toxic quantities of paraquat or diquat. Bipyridyls have large volumes of distribution. Once distribution to tissues has occurred, measures to remove bipyridyls from the blood are very inefficient in reducing the total body burden.

Several strategies are being tested to reduce the frequency of these occurrences. These include the addition of emetics, stenching agents, gelling substances, and bittering agents such as sodim denatonium.

Confirmation of Poisoning: Paraquat and Diquat

At some treatment facilities, a simple colorimetric test is used to identify paraquat and diquat in the urine, and to give a rough indication of the magnitude of absorbed dose. To one volume of urine, add 0.5 volume of freshly prepared 1% sodium dithionite (sodium hydrosulfite) in one normal sodium hydroxide (1.0 N NaOH). Observe color at the end of one minute. A blue color indicates the presence of paraquat in excess of 0.5 mg per liter. Both positive and negative controls should be run to ensure that the dithionite has not undergone oxidation in storage.

When urine collected within 24 hours of paraquat ingestion is tested, the dithionite test appears to have some prognostic value: concentrations less than one milligram per liter (no color to light blue) generally predict survival, while concentrations in excess of one milligram per liter (navy blue to dark blue) often foretell a fatal outcome.

Diquat in urine yields a green color with the dithionite test. Although there is less experience with this test in diquat poisonings, the association of bad prognosis with intense color is probably similar.

Paraquat and diquat can be measured in blood and urine by spectrophotometric, gas chromatographic, liquid chromatographic, and radioimmunoassay methods. These tests are available in numerous clinical reference laboratories and sometimes by the manufacturing company. Survival is likely if plasma concentrations do not exceed 2.0, 0.6, 0.3, 0.16, and 0.1 mg per liter at 4, 6, 10, 16, and 24 hours, respectively, after ingestion.[15]

Treatment

1. Skin and eye decontamination. Flush skin immediately with copious amounts of water. Material splashed in the **eyes** must be removed by **prolonged irrigation** with clean water. Eye contamination should thereafter be treated by an ophthalmologist. Mild skin reactions usually respond if there is no further contact with the pesticide, but the irritation may take several weeks to resolve. Severe injuries with inflammation, cracking, secondary infection, or nail injury should be treated by a dermatologist.

2. Gastrointestinal decontamination. If paraquat or diquat have been ingested, **immediate administration of adsorbent** is the one therapeutic measure most likely to have a favorable effect. **Bentonite** (7.5% suspension) and **Fuller's Earth** (15% suspension) are highly effective, but sometimes not available.

Dosage of Bentonite and Fuller's Earth:

- *Adults and children over 12 years:* 100-150 g.

- *Children under 12 years:* 2 gm/kg body weight.

Caution: Hypercalcemia and fecaliths have sometimes occurred following administration of Fuller's Earth.

Activated charcoal is nearly as effective, and is widely available. See Chapter 2 for dosage of charcoal and further information on gastric decontamination.

Lavage has not been shown to be effective and should not be performed unless the patient is seen within an hour of ingestion. Later lavage runs the risk of inducing bleeding, perforation, or scarring due to additional trauma to already traumatized tissues. Repeated administration of charcoal or other absorbent every 2-4 hours may be beneficial in both children and adults, but use of a cathartic such as sorbitol should be avoided after the first dose. Cathartics and repeat doses of activated charcoal should not be administered if the gut is atonic. **Check frequently for bowel sounds.** Ileus occurs commonly in diquat poisoning, less often in paraquat poisoning.

3. Samples. Secure a blood sample as soon as possible for paraquat analysis, and urine samples for either paraquat and/or diquat. Serial samples of urine for either agent and plasma for paraquat may be followed for prognostic information.

4. Respiration. Do not administer supplemental oxygen until the patient develops severe hypoxemia. High concentrations of oxygen in the lung increase the injury induced by paraquat, and possibly by diquat as well. There may be some advantage in placing the patient in a moderately hypoxic environment, i.e., 15%–16% oxygen, although the benefit of this treatment measure has not been established empirically in human poisonings. Inhalation of nitric oxide has been suggested as a method to maintain tissue oxygenation at low inspired oxygen concentrations, but its efficacy is unproven. When the lung injury is so far advanced that there is no expectation of recovery, oxygen may be given to relieve air hunger.

5. Intensive care. In serious poisonings, care should be provided in an intensive care setting, to allow proper monitoring of body functions and skilled performance of necessary invasive monitoring and procedures.

6. Fluids. It is essential to maintain adequate urinary output.[4] Administer intravenous fluids: isotonic saline, Ringer's solution, or 5% glucose in water. This is highly advantageous early in poisonings as a means of correcting dehydration, accelerating toxicant excretion, reducing tubular fluid concentrations of paraquat, and correcting any metabolic acidosis. However, fluid balance must be monitored carefully to forestall fluid overload if renal failure develops. Monitor the urine regularly for protein and cells, to warn of impending tubular necrosis. Intravenous infusions must be stopped if renal failure occurs, and extracorporeal hemodialysis is indicated. Hemodialysis is not effective in clearing paraquat or diquat from the blood and tissues.

7. Hemoperfusion over cellophane-coated activated charcoal may be considered. The procedure has been used in many paraquat poisonings because the adsorbent does efficiently remove paraquat from the perfused blood. However, recent reviews of effectiveness have failed to show any reduction in mortality as a result of hemoperfusion.[1,4] The apparent reason for this is the very small proportion of paraquat body burden carried in the circulating blood even when only a few hours have elapsed after ingestion. Theoretically, a patient who can be hemoperfused within 10 hours of paraquat ingestion may derive some marginal benefit, but this has not been demonstrated.

If hemoperfusion is attempted, blood calcium and platelet concentrations must be monitored. Calcium and platelets must be replenished if these constituents are depleted by the procedure.

8. Seizure control. Convulsions and psychotic behavior sometimes encountered in diquat poisoning may be best controlled by lorazepam, given slowly intravenously, as outlined in Chapter 2. Control convulsions as outlined in Chapter 2.

9. Other drugs. Many drugs have been tested in animals or given in human bipyridyl poisonings without clear evidence of benefit or harm: corticosteroids, superoxide dismutase, propranolol, cyclophosphamide, vitamin E, riboflavin, niacin, ascorbic acid, clofibrate, desferrioxamine, acetylcysteine, and terpin hydrate. However, recent evidence regarding the use of **cyclophosphamide** and **methylprednisolone** may be effective in reducing the mortality associated with moderate to severe paraquat poisoning. Two studies found a reduced mortality associated with the treatment, while one study found no difference.[16] The dosages used for cyclophosphamide and methylprednisolone were 1 gram daily for two days and 1 gram daily for three days respectively, and were given after hemoperfusion. Each drug was administered as a two hour infusion, and white cell counts, serum creatinine levels, chest radiography, and liver function tests were monitored.[16]

10. Pain management. Morphine sulfate is usually required to control the pain associated with deep mucosal erosions of the mouth, pharynx, and esophagus, as well as abdominal pain from pancreatitis and enteritis. Mouthwashes, cold fluids, ice cream, or anesthetic lozenges may also help to relieve pain in the mouth and throat.

Dosage of Morphine Sulfate:

- *Adults and children over 12 years:* 10-15 mg subcutaneously every 4 hours.

- *Children under 12 years:* 0.1 – 0.2 mg /kg body weight every 4 hours.

---

11. Transplantation. With severe pulmonary toxicity, recovery of the patient may only be accomplished by lung transplantation. However, the transplanted lung is susceptible to subsequent damage due to redistribution of paraquat.[17]

General Chemical Structures

Paraquat

Diquat

References

1. Pond SM. Manifestations and management of paraquat poisoning. *Med J Aust* 1990;152:256-9.

2. Giulivi C, Lavagno CC, Lucesoli F, et al. Lung damage in paraquat poisoning and hyperbaric oxyen exposure: superoxide-mediated inhibition of phospholipase A2. *Free Radic Biol Med* 1995;18:203-13.

3. Nordquist RE, Nguyen H, Poyer JL, et al. The role of free radicals in paraquat-induced corneal lesions. *Free Radic Res* 1995;23:61-71.

4. Honore P, Hantson P, Fauville JP, et al. Paraquat poisoning: State of the art. *Acta Clin Belg* 1994;49:220-8.

5. Bismuth C, Garnier R, Dally S, et al. Prognosis and treatment of paraquat poisoning: A review of 28 cases. *J Toxicol Clin Toxicol* 1982;19:461-74.

6. Harsanyi L, Nemeth A, and Lang A. Paraquat (gramoxone) poisoning in south-west Hungary, 1977-1984. *Am J Forensic Med Pathol* 1987;8:131-4.

7. Lee CC, Lin JL, and Liu L. Recovery of respiratory function in survivors with paraquat intoxication (abstract). *Ann Emerg Med* 1995;26:721-2.

8. Tungsanga K, Chusilp S, Israsena S, et al. Paraquat poisoning: Evidence of systemic toxicity after dermal exposure. *Postgrad Med J* 1983;59:338-9.

9. Vale JA, Meredith TJ, and Buckley BM. Paraquat poisoning: Clinical features and immediate general management. *Hum Toxicol* 1987;6:41-7.

10. Hughes JT. Brain damage due to paraquat poisoning: A fatal case with neuropathological examination of the brain. *Neurotoxicology* 1988;9:243-8.

11. Lam HF, Azawa J, Gupta BN, et al. A comparison of the effects of paraquat and diquat on lung compliance, lung volume, and single-breath diffusing capacity in the rat. *Toxicology* 1980;18:111-23.

12. Vanholder R, Colardyn F, DeReuck J, et al. Diquat intoxication: Report of two cases and review of the literature. *Am J Med* 1981;70:1267-71.

13. Olson KR. Paraquat and diquat. In: Olson KR et al. (eds), Poisoning and Drug Overdose, 2nd ed. Norwalk CT: Appelton and Lange, 1994, pp. 245-6.

14. Sechi GP, Agnetti V, Piredda M, et al. Acute and persistent Parkinsonism after use of diquat. *Neurology* 1992;42:261-3.

15. Proudfoot AT, Stewart MS, Levitt T, et al. Paraquat poisoning: Significance of plasma-paraquat concentrations. *Lancet* 1979;2:330-2.

16. Lin JL, Wei MC, and Liu YC. Pulse therapy with cyclophosphamide and methyprednislone in patients with moderate to severe paraquat poisoning: A preliminary report. *Thorax* 1996;51:661-3.

17. Toronto Lung Transplant Group. Sequential bilateral lung transplantation for paraquat poisoning. A case report. *J Thoracic Cardiovas Surg* 1985;89:734-42.

CHAPTER 13

Other Herbicides

Many herbicides are now available for use in agriculture and for lawn and garden weed control. This chapter discusses herbicides other than the chlorophenoxys, nitrophenols and chlorophenols, arsenicals, and dipyridyls, which are the subjects of separate chapters. Many modern herbicides kill weeds selectively by impairing metabolic processes that are unique to plant life. For this reason, their systemic toxicities in mammals are generally low. Nonetheless, some herbicides pose a significant risk of poisoning if handled carelessly, and many are irritating to eyes, skin, and mucous membranes.

For several good reasons, all of the herbicides mentioned in this chapter should be handled and applied only with full attention to safety measures that minimize personal contact. Many formulations contain adjuvants (stabilizers, penetrants, surfactants) that may have significant irritating and toxic effects. A number of premixed formulations contain two or more active ingredients; the companion pesticides may be more toxic than the principal herbicide. Good hygienic practice should not be disregarded just because a pesticide is reported to have a high LD_{50} in laboratory rodents.

Health professionals who may need to assess the consequences of prior exposure should understand the fate of these compounds after absorption by humans. The water-soluble herbicides are not retained in body tissues for long periods, as were the old lipophilic organochlorine insecticides, such as DDT. Most are excreted, mainly in the urine, within one to four days.

Toxicology

The table on the following pages lists the more commonly used herbicides not discussed elsewhere in this manual. The rat acute oral LD_{50} is given as a rough index of potential lethal toxicity. (If several values are reported by various sources, the lowest is recorded here.) The adverse effect information is drawn from many sources, including product labels, textbooks, published case histories, and some unpublished reports. The listing cannot be considered inclusive, either of herbicide products or of effects.

TOXICITY OF COMMON HERBICIDES

Chemical Class	Generic Name	Proprietary Names	Acute Oral LD$_{50}$ mg/kg	Known or Suspected Adverse Effects
Acetamides	metolachlor	Dual, Pennant, others	2,780	Irritating to eyes and skin.
Aliphatic acids	trichloroacetic acid	TCA	5,000	Irritating to skin, eyes, and respiratory tract.
	dichloropropionic acid (dalapon)	Dalapon, Revenge	970	
Anilides	alachlor	Lasso, Alanox	1,800	Mild irritant.
	propachlor	Ramrod, Bexton, Prolex	710	Dermal irritant and sensitizer.
	propanil	DPA, Chem Rice, Propanex, Riselect, Stam, Stampede	>2,500	Irritating to skin, eyes, and respiratory tract.
Benzamide	pronamide	Kerb, Rapier	8,350	Moderately irritating to eyes
Benzoic, anisic acid derivatives	trichlorobenzoic acid	TCBA, Tribac, 2,3,6-TBA	1,500	Moderately irritating to skin and respiratory tract.
	dicamba	Banvel	2,700	
Benzonitriles	dichlobenil	Casoron, Dyclomec, Barrier	>4,460	Minimal toxic, irritant effects
Benzothiadiazinone dioxide	bentazone	Basagran	>1,000	Irritating to eyes and respiratory tract.
Carbamates and Thiocarbamates (herbicidal)	asulam	Asulox	>5,000	Some are irritating to eyes, skin, and respiratory tract, particularly in concentrated form. Some may be weak inhibitors of cholinesterase.
	terbucarb	Azac, Azar	>34,000	
	butylate	Sutan	3,500	
	cycloate	Ro-Neet	2,000	
	pebulate	Tillam, PEBC	921	
	vernolate	Vernam	1,800	
	EPTC	Eptam, Eradicane	1,630	
	diallate	Di-allate	395	
	triallate	Far-go	1,675	
	thiobencarb	Bolero, Saturn	1,300	

TOXICITY OF COMMON HERBICIDES

Chemical Class	Generic Name	Proprietary Names	Acute Oral LD_{50} mg/kg	Known or Suspected Adverse Effects
Carbanilates	chlorpropham	Sprout-Nip Chloro-IPC	3,800	Skin irritants. May generate methemoglobin at high dosage.
Chloropyridinyl	triclopyr	Garlon, Turflon	630	Irritating to skin and eyes.
Cyclohexenone derivative	sethoxydim	Poast	3,125	Irritating to skin and eyes.
Dinitroamino-benzene derivative	butralin	Amex Tamex	12,600 >5,000	May be moderately irritating. These herbicides do not uncouple oxidative phosphorylation or generate methemoglobin.
	pendimethalin	Prowl, Stomp, Accotab, Herbodox, Go-Go-San, Wax Up	2,250	
	oryzalin	Surflan, Dirimal	>10,000	
Fluorodinitro-toluidine compounds	benfluralin	Benefin, Balan, Balfin, Quilan	>10,000	May be mildly irritating. These herbicides do not uncouple oxidative phosphorylation or generate methemoglobin.
	dinitramine	Cobex	3,000	
	ethalfluralin	Sonalan	>10,000	
	fluchloralin	Basalin	1,550	
	profluralin	Tolban	1,808	
	trifluralin	Treflan	>10,000	
Isoxazolidinone	clomazone	Command	1,369	May be moderately irritating.
Nicotinic acid isopropylamine derivative	imazapyr	Arsenal	>5,000	Irritating to eyes and skin. Does not contain arsenic.
Oxadiazolinone	oxadiazon	Ronstar	>3,500	Minimal toxic and irritant effects.
Phosphonates	glyphosate	Roundup, Glyfonox	4,300	Irritating to eyes, skin, and upper respiratory tract.
	fosamine ammonium	Krenite	>5,000	Irritating to eyes, skin, and upper respiratory tract.

TOXICITY OF COMMON HERBICIDES

Chemical Class	Generic Name	Proprietary Names	Acute Oral LD$_{50}$ mg/kg	Known or Suspected Adverse Effects
Phthalates	chlorthaldimethyl	Dachthal, DCPA	>10,000	Moderately irritating to eyes.
	endothall	Aquathol	51	Free acid is highly toxic. Irritating to skin, eyes and respiratory tract. See Chapter 18.
Picolinic acid compound	picloram	Tordon, Pinene	8,200	Irritating to skin, eyes, and respiratory tract. Low systemic toxicity.
Triazines	ametryn	Ametrex, Evik, Gesapax	1,750	Systemic toxicity is unlikely unless large amounts have been ingested. Some triazines are moderately irritating to the eyes, skin, and respiratory tract.
	atrazine	Aatrex, Atranex, Crisazina	1,780	
	cyanazine	Bladex, Fortrol	288	
	desmetryn	Semeron	1,390	
	metribuzin	Sencor, Lexone, Sencoral, Sencorex	1,100	
	prometryn	Caparol, Gesagard, Prometrex	5.235	
	propazine	Milo-Pro, Primatol, Prozinex	>7,000	
	simazine	Gesatop, Princep, Caliber 90	>5,000	
	terbuthylazine	Gardoprim, Primatol M	2,000	
	tertutryn	Ternit, Prebane, Terbutrex	2,500	
	prometon	Gesafram 50	2,980	
		Pramitol 25E		This particular formulation of prometon is strongly irritating to eyes, skin, and respiratory tract.
Triazole	amitrole, aminotriazole	Amerol, Azolan, Azole, Weedazol	>10,000	Minimal systemic toxicity. Slight irritant effect.

TOXICITY OF COMMON HERBICIDES

Chemical Class	Generic Name	Proprietary Names	Acute Oral LD$_{50}$ mg/kg	Known or Suspected Adverse Effects
Uracils	bromacil	Hyvar	5,200	Irritant to skin, eyes, and respiratory tract. Moderately irritating.
	lenacil	Venzar	>11,000	
	terabacil	Sinbar	>5,000	
Urea derivatives	chlorimuron ethyl	Classic	>4,000	Systemic toxicity is unlikely unless large amounts have been ingested.
	chlorotoluron	Dicuran, Tolurex	>10,000	
	diuron	Cekiuron, Crisuron, Dailon, Direx, Diurex, Diuron, Karmex, Unidron, Vonduron	>5,000	Many substituted ureas are irritating to eyes, skin, and mucous membranes.
	flumeturon	Cotoran, cottonex	8,900	
	isoproturon	Alon, Arelon, IP50, Tolkan	1,826	
	linuron	Afalon, Linex, Linorox, Linurex, Lorox, Sarclex	1,500	
	methabenz-thiazuron	Tribunil	5,000	
	metobromuron	Pattonex	2,000	
	metoxuron	Deftor, Dosaflo, Purivel, Sulerex	3,200	
	monolinuron	Aresin	2,100	
	monuron	Monuron	3,600	
	neburon	Granurex, Neburex	>11,000	
	siduron	Tupersan	>7,500	
	sulfemeturon-methyl	Oust	>5,000	
	tebuthiuron	Spike, Tebusan	644	

Confirmation of Poisoning

Although there are analytical methods for residues of many of the herbicides mentioned in this chapter and for some of the mammalian metabolites generated from them, these procedures are not generally available to confirm human absorption of the chemicals. Exposure must be determined from a recent history of occupational contact or accidental or deliberate ingestion.

Treatment

1. Skin decontamination. Skin contamination should be treated promptly by washing with soap and water. Contamination of the eyes should be treated immediately by prolonged flushing of the eyes with large amounts of clean water. If dermal or ocular irritation persists, medical attention should be obtained without delay. See Chapter 2.

2. Gastrointestinal decontamination. Ingestions of these herbicides are likely to be followed by vomiting and diarrhea due to their irritant properties. Management depends on: (1) the best estimate of the quantity ingested, (2) time elapsed since ingestion, and (3) the clinical status of the subject.

Activated charcoal is probably effective in limiting irritant effects and reducing absorption of most or all of these herbicides. Aluminum hydroxide antacids may be useful in neutralizing the irritant actions of more acidic agents. Sorbitol should be given to induce catharsis if bowel sounds are present and if spontaneous diarrhea has not already commenced. Dehydration and electrolyte disturbances may be severe enough to require oral or intravenous fluids.

There are no specific antidotes for poisoning by these herbicides. In the case of suicidal ingestions, particularly, the possibility must always be kept in mind that multiple toxic substances may have been swallowed.

If large amounts of herbicide have been ingested and the patient is seen within an hour of the ingestion, gastrointestinal decontamination should be considered, as outlined in Chapter 2.

If the amount of ingested herbicides was small, if effective emesis has already occurred, or if treatment is delayed, administer activated charcoal and sorbitol by mouth.

3. Intravenous fluids. If serious dehydration and electrolyte depletion have occurred as a result of vomiting and diarrhea, monitor blood electrolytes and fluid balance and administer intravenous infusions of glucose, normal saline, Ringer's solution, or Ringer's lactate to restore extracellular fluid volume and electrolytes. Follow this with oral nutrients as soon as fluids can be retained.

4. Supportive measures are ordinarily sufficient for successful management of excessive exposures to these herbicides (endothall is an exception—see Chapter 18, p. 187). If the patient's condition deteriorates in spite of good supportive care, the operation of an alternative or additional toxicant should be suspected.

Section IV

OTHER PESTICIDES

Arsenical Pesticides

Many arsenic compounds have been discontinued in the United States as a result of government regulations. However, arsenical pesticides are still widely available in some countries, and many homes and farms have leftover supplies that continue to represent some residual risk.

Arsine gas is discussed separately on page 132.

Toxicology

Arsenic is a natural element that has both metal and nonmetal physical/chemical properties. In some respects, it resembles nitrogen, phosphorus, antimony, and bismuth in its chemical behavior. In nature, it exists in elemental, trivalent (-3 or +3), and pentavalent (+5) states. It binds covalently with most nonmetals (notably oxygen and sulfur) and with metals (for example, calcium and lead). It forms stable trivalent and pentavalent organic compounds. In biochemical behavior, it resembles phosphorus, competing with phosphorus analogs for chemical binding sites.

Toxicity of the various arsenic compounds in mammals extends over a wide range, determined in part by the unique biochemical actions of each compound, but also by absorbability and efficiency of biotransformation and disposition. Overall, arsines present the greatest toxic hazard, followed closely by arsenites (inorganic trivalent compounds). Inorganic pentavalent compounds (arsenates) are somewhat less toxic than arsenites, while the organic (methylated) pentavalent compounds represent the least hazard of the arsenicals that are used as pesticides.[1]

The pentavalent arsenicals are relatively water soluble and absorbable across mucous membranes. Trivalent arsenicals, having greater lipid solubility, are more readily absorbed across the skin.[2] However, poisonings by dermal absorption of either form have been extremely rare. Ingestion has been the usual basis of poisoning; gut absorption efficiency depends on the physical form of the compound, its solubility characteristics, the gastric pH, gastrointestinal motility, and gut microbial transformation. Arsine exposure occurs primarily through inhalation, and toxic effects may also occur with other arsenicals through inhalation of aerosols.

Once absorbed, many arsenicals cause toxic injury to cells of the nervous system, blood vessels, liver, kidney, and other tissues. Two biochemical mechanisms of toxicity are recognized: (1) reversible combination with thiol groups contained in tissue proteins and enzymes, and (2) substitution of arsenic anions for phosphate in many reactions, including those critical to oxidative phosphorylation. Arsenic is readily metabolized in the kidney to a methylated form, which is much less toxic and easily excreted. However, it is generally safest to manage cases of arsenical pesticide ingestion as though all forms are highly toxic.

The unique toxicology of arsine gas is described later in this chapter.

Signs and Symptoms of Poisoning

Manifestations of acute poisoning are distinguishable from those of chronic poisoning.

Acute arsenic poisoning: Symptoms and signs usually appear within one hour after ingestion, but may be delayed several hours. Garlic odor of the breath and feces may help to identify the toxicant in a severely poisoned patient. There is often a metallic taste in the mouth. Adverse gastrointestinal (GI) effects predominate, with vomiting, abdominal pain, and rice-water or bloody diarrhea being the most common. Other GI effects include inflammation, vesicle formation and eventual sloughing of the mucosa in the mouth, pharynx, and esophagus.[3] These effects result from the action of an arsenical metabolite on blood vessels generally, and the splanchnic vasculature in particular, causing dilation and increased capillary permeability.

The central nervous system is also commonly affected during acute exposure. Symptoms may begin with headache, dizziness, drowsiness, and confusion. Symptoms may progress to include muscle weakness and spasms, hypothermia, lethargy, delirium, coma, and convulsions.[1] Renal injury is manifest as proteinuria, hematuria, glycosuria, oliguria, casts in the urine, and, in severe poisoning, acute tubular necrosis. Cardiovascular manifestations include shock, cyanosis, and cardiac arrhythmia,[4,5] which are due to direct toxic action and electrolyte disturbances. Liver damage may be manifested by elevated liver enzymes and jaundice. Injury to blood-forming tissues may cause anemia, leukopenia, and thrombocytopenia.

Death usually occurs one to three days following onset of symptoms and is often the result of circulatory failure, although renal failure also may contribute.[1] If the patient survives, painful paresthesias, tingling, and numbness in the hands and feet may be experienced as a delayed sequela of acute exposure. This sensorimotor peripheral neuropathy, which may include muscle weakness and spasms, typically begins 1–3 weeks after exposure.[6] The muscle weakness may be confused with Guillain-Barre syndrome.[7]

Chronic arsenic poisoning from repeated absorption of toxic amounts generally has an insidious onset of clinical effects and may be difficult to diagnose. Neurologic, dermal, and nonspecific manifestations are usually more prominent than the gastrointestinal effects that characterize acute poisoning. Muscle

Commercial Products

(Many have been discontinued)

arsenic acid
  Hi-Yield Dessicant H-10
  Zotox
arsenic trioxide
cacodylic acid (sodium cacodylate)
  Bolate
  Bolls-Eye
  Bophy
  Dilie
  Kack
  Phytar 560
  Rad-E-Cate 25
  Salvo
calcium acid methane arsonate (CAMA)
  Calar
  Super Crab-E-Rad-Calar
  Super Dal-E-Rad
calcium arsenate
  Spra-cal
  tricalcium arsenate
  Turf-Cal
calcium arsenite
  London purple
  mono-calcium arsenite
copper acetoarsenite
  Emerald green
  French green
  Mitis green
  Paris green
  Schweinfurt green
copper arsenite (acid copper arsenite)
disodium methane arsonate
  Ansar 8100
  Arrhenal
  Arsinyl
  Crab-E-Rad
  Di-Tac
  DMA
  DSMA
  Methar 30
  Sodar
  Weed-E-Rad 360
lead arsenate
  Gypsine
  Soprabel
methane arsonic acid (MAA)
monoammonium methane arsonate (MAMA)
monosodium methane arsonate (MSMA)
  Ansar 170

(Continued on the next page)

weakness and fatigue can occur, as can anorexia and weight loss. Hyperpigmentation is a common sign, and tends to be accentuated in areas that are already more pigmented, such as the groin and areola. Hyperkeratosis is another very common sign, especially on the palms and soles.[8,9] Subcutaneous edema of the face, eyelids, and ankles, stomatitis, white striations across the nails (Mees lines), and sometimes loss of nails or hair are other signs of chronic, continuous exposure.[1,9] On occasion, these hyperkeratotic papules have undergone malignant transformation.[8] Years after exposure, dermatologic findings include squamous cell and basal cell carcinoma, often in sun-protected areas.

Neurologic symptoms are also common with chronic exposure. Peripheral neuropathy, manifested by paresthesia, pain, anesthesia, paresis, and ataxia, may be a prominent feature. It may often begin with sensory symptoms in the lower extremities and progress to muscular weakness and eventually paralysis and muscle wasting. Although less common, encephalopathy can develop with speech and mental disturbances very much like those seen in thiamine deficiency (Wernicke's syndrome).

Other organ systems are affected with arsenic toxicity. Liver injury reflected in hepatomegaly and jaundice may progress to cirrhosis, portal hypertension, and ascites. Arsenic has direct glomerular and tubular toxicity resulting in oliguria, proteinuria, and hematuria. Electrocardiographic abnormalities (prolongation of the Q-T interval) and peripheral vascular disease have been reported. The latter includes acrocyanosis, Raynaud's phenomenon, and frank gangrene.[1,10] Hematologic abnormalities include anemia, leukopenia, and thrombocytopenia.[1] Late sequelae of protracted high intakes of arsenic include skin cancer as described above and an increased risk of lung cancer.[1,8]

Confirmation of Poisoning

Measurement of 24-hour urinary excretion of arsenic (micrograms per day) is the most common way to confirm excessive absorption and is the preferred method to follow serial levels and evaluate chronic exposure.[1,11] Spot urine arsenic analysis expressed as a ratio with urinary creatinine is the recommended method to evaluate occupational exposures.[12] Methods to determine blood arsenic concentration are available; however blood levels tend to poorly correlate with exposure except in the initial acute phase.[11,13] Special metal-free acid-washed containers should be used for sample collection. Arsenic excretion above 100 mcg per day should be viewed with suspicion and the test should be repeated.

Excretions above 200 mcg per day reflect a toxic intake, unless seafood was ingested.[11,13,14,15] Diets rich in seafood, primarily shellfish in the previous 48 hours, may generate 24-hour urine excretion levels as high as 200 mcg per day and sometimes more.[3,14] The majority of marine arsenic that is excreted is in the methylated form (arsenobetaine) and is not considered acutely toxic. However, a recent study supports that some of the arsenic released from mussels may contain higher amounts of arsenic trioxide than previously thought.[14] Urinary arsenic may be speciated into inorganic and organic fractions to help determine the source of the exposure and to help guide treatment.

Concentrations of arsenic in blood, urine, or other biologic materials can be measured by either wet or dry ashing, followed by colorimetric or atomic absorption spectrometric analysis. The latter method is preferred. Blood concentrations in excess of about 100 mcg per liter probably indicate excessive intake or occupational exposure, provided that seafood was not ingested before the sample was taken.[3,11,13,15] Blood samples tend to correlate with urine samples during the early stages of acute ingestion,[11] but because arsenic is rapidly cleared from the blood, the 24-hour urine sample remains the preferred method for detection and for ongoing monitoring.[1,11,13] Hair has been used for evaluation of chronic exposure. Levels in unexposed people are usually less than 1 mg/kg; levels in individuals with chronic poisoning range between 1 and 5 mg/kg.[15] Hair samples should be viewed with caution because external environmental contamination such as air pollution may artificially elevate arsenic levels.

Special tests for arsine toxicosis are described on page 132 under "Arsine Gas."

Treatment

The following discussion applies principally to poisonings by arsenicals in solid or dissolved form. Treatment of poisoning by arsine gas requires special measures described below on page 132.

1. Skin decontamination. Wash arsenical pesticide from skin and hair with copious amounts of soap and water. Flush contaminant from eyes with clean water. If irritation persists, specialized medical treatment should be obtained. See Chapter 2.

2. Gastrointestinal decontamination. If arsenical pesticide has been ingested within the first hour of treatment, consideration should be given to GI decontamination, as outlined in Chapter 2. Because poisoning by ingested arsenic almost always results in profuse diarrhea, it is generally not appropriate to administer a cathartic.

3. Intravenous fluids. Administer intravenous fluids to restore adequate hydration, support urine flow, and correct electrolyte imbalances. Monitor intake/output continuously to guard against fluid overload. If acute renal failure occurs, monitor blood electrolytes regularly. Blood transfusions and oxygen by mask may be needed to combat shock.

4. Cardiopulmonary monitoring. Monitor cardiac status by ECG to detect ventricular arrhythmias including prolonged Q-T interval and ventricular tachycardia, and toxic myocardiopathy (T wave inversion, long S-T interval).

5. Chelation therapy. Administration of Dimercaprol (BAL) is usually indicated in symptomatic arsenic poisonings, although DMPS, where available, may prove to be a better antidote. The following dosage schedule has proven to be effective in accelerating arsenic excretion.

Monitor urinary arsenic excretion while any chelating agent is being administered. When 24-hour excretion falls below 50 mcg per day, it usually is advisable to discontinue the chelation therapy.

RECOMMENDED INTRAMUSCULAR DOSAGE OF BAL (DIMERCAPROL) IN ARSENIC POISONING

	Severe Poisoning	Mild Poisoning
1st day	3.0 mg/kg q4h (6 injections)	2.5 mg/kg q6h (4 injections)
2nd day	3.0 mg/kg q4h (6 injections)	2.5 mg/kg q6h (4 injections)
3rd day	3.0 mg/kg q6h (4 injections)	2.5 mg/kg q12h (2 injections)
Each of the following days for 10 days, or until recovery	3.0 mg/kg q12 hr (2 injections)	2.5 mg/kg qd (1 injection)

BAL is provided as a 100 mg/mL solution in oil. Dosages in the table are in terms of BAL itself, not of the solution. Dosages for children are consistent with the "Mild Poisoning" schedule and can be between 2.5 and 3.0 mg/kg per dose.[16]

Caution: Disagreeable side effects often accompany the use of BAL: nausea, headache, burning and tingling sensations, sweating, pain in the back and abdomen, tremor, restlessness, tachycardia, hypertension, and fever. Coma and convulsions occur at very high dosage. Sterile abscesses may form at injection sites. Acute symptoms usually subside in 30-90 minutes. Antihistamine drugs or an oral dose of 25-50 mg ephedrine sulfate or pseudoephedrine provide relief. These are more effective if given a few minutes before the injection of BAL. BAL may potentially have other adverse effects. In rabbits, treatment of arsenite exposure with BAL increased brain arsenic levels.[17]

6. Oral treatments. After the gastrointestinal tract is reasonably free of arsenic, oral administration of d-penicillamine, Succimer (DMSA), or DMPS should probably replace BAL therapy. However, d-penicillamine has demonstrated limited effectiveness for arsenic exposure in experimental models.[18]

> **Dosage of d-penicillamine:**
>
> - *Adults and children over 12 years:* 0.5 g every 6 hours, given 30–60 minutes before meals and at bedtime for about 5 days.
>
> - *Children under 12 years:* 0.1 g/kg body weight, every 6 hours, given 30–60 minutes before meals and at bedtime for about 5 days. Not to exceed 1.0 g per day.
>
> **Caution:** Adverse reactions to short-term therapy are rare. However, **persons allergic to penicillin should not receive d-penicillamine** as they may suffer allergic reactions to it.

Succimer (DMSA) has been shown to be an effective chelator of arsenic, though it is not labeled for this indication.[19] In Europe, DMPS has been used successfully in treatment of arsenic poisoning. In light of the lack of effectiveness of d-penicillamine, coupled with the low toxicity and high therapeutic index of DMPS and DMSA, it appears that the latter two agents may be the preferred method for chronic toxicity or when oral chelation is acceptable.[18,19]

> **Dosage of DMSA (Succimer):**
>
> - *Adults and Children:* 10 mg/kg every 8 hours for 5 days, followed by 10 mg/kg every 12 hours for an additional 14 days. (Maximum 500 mg per dose). Should be given with food.
>
> **Dosage of DMPS:**
>
> - *Adults:* 100 mg every 8 hours for 3 weeks to 9 months.

7. Hemodialysis. Extracorporeal hemodialysis, used in combination with BAL therapy, has limited effectiveness in removing arsenic from the blood. Hemodialysis is clearly indicated to enhance arsenic elimination and maintain extracellular fluid composition if acute renal failure occurs.

8. Renal function. In patients with intact renal function, alkalinization of the urine by sodium bicarbonate to maintain urine pH >7.5 may help protect renal function in the face of hemolysis occurring as part of the acute poisoning.

HIGHLIGHTS

• Powerful hemolysin

Signs and Symptoms:

• Malaise, dizziness, nausea, abdominal pain

• Hemoglobinuria and jaundice.

Treatment:

• Supportive

• Exchange transfusion may be considered

ARSINE GAS

Arsine is not used as a pesticide. However, some poisonings by arsine have occurred in pesticide manufacturing plants and metal refining operations when arsenicals came into contact with mineral acids or strong reducing agents.

Toxicology

Arsine is a powerful **hemolysin,** a toxic action not exhibited by other arsenicals. In some individuals, very little inhalation exposure is required to cause a serious hemolytic reaction. Exposure times of 30 minutes at 25-50 parts per million are considered lethal.[20] Symptoms of poisoning usually appear 1-24 hours after exposure: headache, malaise, weakness, dizziness, dyspnea, nausea, abdominal pain, and vomiting. Dark red urine (hemoglobinuria) is often passed 4-6 hours after exposure. Usually 1-2 days after hemoglobinuria appears, jaundice is evident. Hemolytic anemia, sometimes profound, usually provides diagnostic confirmation and can cause severe weakness. Abdominal tenderness and liver enlargement are often apparent. Basophilic stippling of red cells, red cell fragments, and ghosts are seen in the blood smear. Methemoglobinemia and methemoglobinuria are evident. Elevated concentrations of arsenic are found in the urine, but these are not nearly as high as are found in poisonings by solid arsenicals. Plasma content of unconjugated bilirubin is elevated.

Renal failure due to direct toxic action of arsine and to products of hemolysis represents the chief threat to life in arsine poisoning.[21]

Polyneuropathy and a mild psycho-organic syndrome are reported to have followed arsine intoxication after a latency of 1-6 months.

Treatment

1. Remove the victim to fresh air.

2. Administer intravenous fluids to keep the urine as dilute as possible and to support excretion of arsenic and products of hemolysis. Include sufficient sodium bicarbonate to keep the urine alkaline (pH greater than 7.5).

Caution: Monitor fluid balance carefully to avoid fluid overload if renal failure supervenes. Monitor plasma electrolytes to detect disturbances (particularly hyperkalemia) as early as possible.

3. Monitor urinary arsenic excretion to assess severity of poisoning. The amount of arsine that must be absorbed to cause poisoning is small, and therefore high levels of urinary arsenic excretion may not always occur, even in the face of significant poisoning.[21,22]

4. If poisoning is severe, exchange blood transfusion may be considered. It was successful in rescuing one adult victim of arsine poisoning.

5. Extracorporeal hemodialysis may be necessary to maintain normal extracellular fluid composition and to enhance arsenic elimination if renal failure occurs, but it is not very effective in removing arsine carried in the blood.

General Chemical Structures

INORGANIC TRIVALENT

Arsenic trioxide

$$As - O - As$$ with O above and O below

"White arsenic." Arsenous oxide. Has been discontinued but still may be available from prior registrations.

Sodium arsenite

$$Na - O - As = O$$

Sodanit, Prodalumnol Double. All uses discontinued in the U.S.

Calcium arsenite

$$O - As = O$$
$$Ca \text{ (approx.)}$$
$$O - As = O$$

Mono-calcium arsenite, London purple. Flowable powder for insecticidal use on fruit. All uses discontinued in the U.S.

Copper arsenite
(Acid copper arsenite)

$$HO - Cu - O - As = O$$

Wettable powder, for use as insecticide, wood preservative. All uses discontinued in the U.S.

Copper acetoarsenite

$$Cu - (O - C - CH_3)_2$$ with O double-bonded to C
$$3Cu - (O - As = O)_2$$

Insecticide. Paris green, Schweinfurt green, Emerald green, French green, Mitis green. No longer used in the U.S.; still used outside U.S.

Arsine

$$As$$ with H, H, H

Not a pesticide. Occasionally generated during manufacture of arsenicals.

INORGANIC PENTAVALENT

Arsenic acid

$$HO, OH$$
$$As = O$$
$$HO$$

Hi-Yield Dessicant H-10, Zotox. Water solutions used as defoliants, herbicides, and wood preservatives.

Sodium arsenate

$$NaO, OH$$
$$As = O$$
$$NaO$$

Disodium arsenate. Jones Ant Killer. All uses discontinued, but may still be encountered from old registration.

Calcium arsenate	Tricalcium arsenate, Spra-cal, Turf-Cal. Flowable powder formulations used against weeds, grubs. No longer used in the U.S.
Lead arsenate	Gypsine, Soprabel. Limited use in the U.S.; wettable powder used as insecticide outside the U.S.
Zinc arsenate	Powder once used in U.S. as insecticide on potatoes and tomatoes.

ORGANIC (PENTAVALENT)

Cacodylic acid (sodium cacodylate) (or Na)	Non-selective herbicide, defoliant, silvicide. Bolate, Bolls-Eye, Bophy, Dilic, Kack, Phytar 560, Rad-E-Cate 25, Salvo.
Methane arsonic acid	MAA. Non-selective herbicide.
Monosodium methane arsonate	MSMA. Non-selective herbicide, defoliant, silvicide. Ansar 170, Arsonate Liquid, Bueno 6, Daconate 6, Dal-E-Rad, Drexar 530, Herbi-All, Merge 823, Mesamate, Target MSMA, Trans-Vert, Weed-E-Rad, Weed-Hoe.
Disodium methane arsonate	DSMA. Selective post-emergence herbicide, silvicide. Ansar 8100, Arrhenal, Arsinyl, Crab-E-Rad, Di-Tac, DMA, Methar 30, Sodar, Weed-E-Rad 360.
Monoammonium methane arsonate	MAMA. Selective post-emergence herbicide. No longer used in the U.S.

Calcium acid methane arsonate

$$CH_3 \quad OH \qquad HO \quad CH_3$$
$$\backslash As / \qquad \backslash As /$$
$$O \diagup\!\!\!\!= \quad O - Ca - O \qquad O$$

CAMA. Selective post-emergence herbicide. Calar, Super Crab-E-Rad-Calar, Super Dal-E-Rad.

References

1. Malachowski ME. An update on arsenic. *Clin Lab Med* 1990; 10(3):459-72.

2. Ellenhorn, MJ. Arsenic: Metals and related compounds. In: Ellenhorn's Medical Toxicology, Diagnosis and Treatment of Human Poisoning, 2nd ed. Baltimore: Williams & Wilkins, 1997, p. 1540.

3. Campbell JP and Alvarez JA. Acute arsenic intoxication. *Am Fam Physician* 1989; 40(6):93-7.

4. St. Petery J, Gross C, and Victorica BE. Ventricular fibrillation caused by arsenic poisoning. *AJDC* 1970;120:367-71.

5. Goldsmith S and From AHL. Arsenic-induced atypical ventricular tachycardia. *New Engl J Med* 1980; 303(19).1096-8.

6. Heyman A, Pfeiffer JB Jr., Willett RW, et al. Peripheral neuropathy caused by arsenical intoxication. A study of 41 cases with observations on the effects of BAL (2,3-dimercapto-propanol). *N Engl J Med* 1956;254:401-9.

7. Donofrio PD, Wilbourn AJ, Albers JW, et al. Acute arsenic intoxication presenting as Guillain-Barre-like syndrome. *Muscle Nerve* 1987; 10:114-20.

8. Maloney ME. Arsenic in dermatology. *Dermatol Surg* 1996;22:301-4.

9. Navarro B, Sayas MJ, Atienza A, and León P. An unhappily married man with thick soles. *Lancet* 1996;347:1596.

10. Lin TH, Huang YL, and Wang MY. Arsenic species in drinking water, hair, fingernails, and urine of patients with blackfoot disease. *J Toxicol Environ Health* 1998;53A:85-93.

11. Fesmire FM, Schauben JL, and Roberge RJ. Survival following massive arsenic ingestion. *Am J Emerg Med,* 1998;6(6):602-6.

12. ACGIH. 1997 TLVs and BEIs. Threshold limit values for chemical substances and physical agents. Biological exposure indices. Cincinnati, 1997.

13. Wagner SL and Weswig P. Arsenic in blood and urine of forest workers. *Arch Environ Health* 1974; 28:77-9.

14. Buchet JP, Pauwels J, and Lauwerys R. Assessment of exposure to inorganic arsenic following ingestion of marine organisms by volunteers. *Environ Res* 1994;66:44-51.

15. Baselt RA and Cravey RH. Arsenic. In: Disposition of Toxic Drugs and Chemicals in Men, 3rd ed. Chicago, IL: Year Book Medical Publishers, 1990, pp. 65-9.

16. Barone MA. Drug doses; Dimercaprol. In: The Harriet Lane Handbook, 14th ed. Baltimore: Mosby, 1996, p. 525.

17. Hoover TD and Aposhian HV. BAL increased the arsenic-74 content of rabbit brain. *Toxicol Appl Pharmacol* 1983; 70:160-2.

18. Kreppel H, Reichl FX, Forth W, and Fichtl B. Lack of effectiveness of d–penicillamine in experimental arsenic poisoning. *Vet Hum Toxicol* 1989;31:1-5.

19. Mückter H, Liebl B, Beichl FX, et al. Are we ready to replace dimercaprol (BAL) as an arsenic antidote? *Hum Exp Toxicol* 1997;16:460-5.

20. Blackwell M and Robbins A. NIOSH Current Intelligence Bulletin #32, Arsine (arsenic hydride) poisoning in the workplace. *Am Ind Hyg Assoc J* 1979;40:A56-61.

21. Fowler BA and Weissberg JB. Arsine poisoning. *New Engl J Med* 1974;291:1171-4.

22. Rathus E, Stingon RG, and Putman JL. Arsine poisoning, country style. *Med J Aust* 1979;1:163-6.

CHAPTER 15

Fungicides

Fungicides are extensively used in industry, agriculture, and the home and garden for a number of purposes, including: protection of seed grain during storage, shipment, and germination; protection of mature crops, berries, seedlings, flowers, and grasses in the field, in storage, and during shipment; suppression of mildews that attack painted surfaces; control of slime in paper pulps; and protection of carpet and fabrics in the home.

Fungicides vary enormously in their potential for causing adverse effects in humans. Historically, some of the most tragic epidemics of pesticide poisoning occurred because of mistaken consumption of seed grain treated with organic mercury or hexachlorobenzene. However, most fungicides currently in use are unlikely to cause frequent or severe systemic poisonings for several reasons. First, many have low inherent toxicity in mammals and are inefficiently absorbed. Second, many fungicides are formulated as suspensions of wettable powders or granules, from which rapid, efficient absorption is unlikely. And third, methods of application are such that relatively few individuals are intensively exposed. Apart from systemic poisonings, fungicides as a class are probably responsible for a disproportionate number of irritant injuries to skin and mucous membranes, as well as dermal sensitization.

The following discussion covers the recognized adverse effects of widely used fungicides. For fungicides that have caused systemic poisoning, recommendations for management of poisonings and injuries are set forth. For fungicides not known to have caused systemic poisonings in the past, only general guidelines can be offered.

The discussion of fungicide-related adverse effects proceeds in this order:

- Substituted Benzenes
- Thiocarbamates
- Ethylene Bis Dithiocarbamates
- Thiophthalimides
- Copper Compounds
- Organomercury Compounds
- Organotin Compounds
- Cadmium Compounds
- Miscellaneous Organic Fungicides

HIGHLIGHTS

- Numerous fungicides in use with varying levels of toxicity
- Other than organomercury compounds, most fungicides are unlikely to be absorbed enough to cause systemic poisonings

Signs and Symptoms:

- Variable

Treatment:

- Dermal and eye decontamination
- GI decontamination
- Intravenous fluids

Contraindicated:

- Atropine. Fungicides are not cholinesterase inhibitors

SUBSTITUTED BENZENES

Toxicology

Chloroneb is supplied as wettable powder for treatment of soil and seed. This agent exhibits very low oral toxicity in mammals. It may be moderately irritating to skin and mucous membranes. The metabolite dichloromethoxyphenol is excreted in the urine. No cases of systemic poisoning in humans have been reported.

Chlorothalonil is available as wettable powder, water dispersible granules, and flowable powders. Chlorothalonil has caused irritation of skin and mucous membranes of the eye and respiratory tract on contact. Cases of allergic contact dermatitis have been reported. There is one report of immediate anaphylactoid reaction to skin contact.[1] It is apparently poorly absorbed across the skin and the gastrointestinal lining. No cases of systemic poisoning in humans have been reported.

Dicloran is a broad-spectrum fungicide widely used to protect perishable produce. It is formulated as wettable powder, dusts, and flowable powders. Dicloran is absorbed by occupationally exposed workers, but it is promptly eliminated, at least partly in the urine. Biotransformation products include dichloroaminophenol, which is an uncoupler of oxidative phosphorylation (enhances heat production). Extraordinary doses of dicloran given to laboratory animals cause liver injury and corneal opacities.

Based on laboratory animal studies and effects of similar compounds, large doses might be expected to cause liver injury, pyrexia, corneal opacities, and possibly methemoglobinemia. None of these have been observed in humans exposed to DCNA.

Hexachlorobenzene. Principal formulations are dusts and powders. Hexachlorobenzene differs chemically and toxicologically from hexachlorocyclohexane, the gamma isomer of which (lindane) is still a widely-used insecticide.

Although this seed protectant fungicide has only slight irritant effects and relatively low single-dose toxicity, long-term ingestion of HCB-treated grain by Turkish farm dwellers in the late 1950s caused several thousand cases of toxic porphyria resembling porphyria cutanea tarda.[2] This condition was due to impaired hemoglobin synthesis, leading to toxic end-products (porphyrins) in body tissues. The disease was characterized by excretion of red-tinged (porphyrin-containing) urine, bullous lesions of light-exposed skin, scarring and atrophy of skin with overgrowth of hair, liver enlargement, loss of appetite, arthritic disease, and wasting of skeletal muscle mass. Although most adults ultimately recovered after they stopped consuming the HCB-treated grain, some infants nursed by affected mothers died.

Hexachlorobenzene is effectively dechlorinated and oxidized in humans; trichlorophenols are the major urinary excretion products. Disposition is sufficiently prompt that occupationally exposed workers usually show only slight elevation of blood HCB concentrations. HCB is sometimes present in blood specimens from "non-occupationally exposed" persons in concentrations of up to 5 mcg per liter. Residues in food are the probable cause.

Pentachloronitrobenzene is used to dress seed and treat soil. Formulations include emulsifiable concentrates, wettable powders, and granules. Hexachlorobenzene is a minor contaminant to technical PCNB.

High concentrations in prolonged contact with skin have caused sensitization in some tested volunteers, but neither irritation nor sensitization has been reported in occupationally exposed workers. One case of conjunctivitis and keratitis occurred following eye contamination. This resolved slowly but completely.

Systemic poisonings have not been reported. Clearance in laboratory animals is slow, probably due to enterohepatic recirculation. Excretion is chiefly biliary, with some conversion to pentachloroaniline, pentachlorophenol, and other metabolites in the liver. Although a methemoglobinemic effect might be suspected (as from nitrobenzene), this has not been reported in humans or animals, nor has toxic porphyria (as from hexachlorobenzene) been reported.

Confirmation of Poisoning

Hexachlorobenzene (HCB) can be measured in blood by gas chromatography. Chlorophenol metabolites can be measured in the urine. Although inherited disease and a number of exogenous agents may cause porphyrins to appear in the urine, a test for porphyrins may be useful for toxicological diagnosis if there has been a known exposure to HCB or if a patient exhibits signs suggestive of porphyria cutanea tarda.

Gas chromatography can be used to measure PCNB and metabolites, chlorothalonil, and chloroneb, but the analysis is not widely available. Methods have also been described for analysis of dicloran, but they are not widely available.

Treatment

1. Skin decontamination. Dermal contamination should be washed off with soap and water. Flush contamination from the eyes with copious amounts of water. If irritation persists, specialized medical care should be obtained. See Chapter 2.

2. Gastrointestinal decontamination. If a large amount of the fungicide has been ingested in the last few hours, and if copious vomiting has not already occurred, it may be reasonable to consider GI decontamination. Activated charcoal can be used along with the addition of the cathartic sorbitol to the charcoal slurry. If sorbitol is given separately, it should be diluted with an equal volume of water before administration. No more than one dose of sorbitol is recommended and it should be used with caution in children and the elderly. See Chapter 2 for appropriate dosages.

If contact with the toxicant has been minimal (for example, oral contamination only, promptly flushed out of the mouth), administration of charcoal without a cathartic, followed by careful observation of the patient, probably represents optimal management.

3. Porphyria. Persons affected by porphyria should avoid sunlight, which exacerbates the dermal injury by porphyrins.

THIOCARBAMATES

Thiocarbamates are commonly formulated as dusts, wettable powders, or water suspensions. They are used to protect seeds, seedlings, ornamentals, turf, vegetables, fruit, and apples. Unlike the N-methyl carbamates (Chapter 5), thiocarbamates have very little insecticidal potency. A few exhibit weak anticholinesterase activity, but most have no significant effect on this enzyme. Overall, they are less of a threat to human health than the insecticidal carbamates. Fungicidal thiocarbamates are discussed in this section, while those used as herbicides are considered in Chapter 13.

METAM-SODIUM

Metam-sodium is formulated in aqueous solutions for application as a soil biocide and fumigant to kill fungi, bacteria, weed seeds, nematodes, and insects. All homeowner uses have been cancelled in the United States.

Toxicology

Metam-sodium can be very irritating to the skin. Poisonings by ingestion of metam-sodium have not been reported. Although animal feeding studies do not indicate extraordinary toxicity of metam-sodium by ingestion, its decomposition in water yields methyl isothiocyanate, a gas that is extremely irritating to respiratory mucous membranes, to the eyes, and to the lungs. Inhalation of methyl isothiocyanate may cause pulmonary edema (severe respiratory distress, coughing of bloody, frothy sputum). For this reason, metam-sodium is considered a fumigant. It must be used in outdoor settings only, and stringent precautions must be taken to avoid inhalation of evolved gas.

Theoretically, exposure to metam-sodium may predispose the individual to Antabuse reactions if alcohol is ingested after exposure. (See Thiram.) However, no such occurrences have been reported.

Confirmation of Poisoining

No tests for metam–sodium or its breakdown products in body fluids are available.

Treatment

1. Skin decontamination. Skin contamination should be washed off with soap and water. Flush contamination from the eyes with copious amounts of water to avoid burns and corneal injury. If dermal or eye irritation persists, specialized medical treatment should be obtained. See Chapter 2.

2. Gastrointestinal decontamination. If a large amount has been ingested recently, consider gastric emptying or charcoal and cathartic. See Chapter 2 for appropriate dosages.

3. Pulmonary edema. If pulmonary irritation or edema occur as a result of inhaling methyl isothiocyanate, transport the victim promptly to a medical facility. Treatment for pulmonary edema should proceed as outlined in Chapter 16, Fumigants.

4. Contraindicated: Metam-sodium is not a cholinesterase inhibitor. Atropine is not an antidote.

THIRAM

Thiram is a common component of latex and possibly responsible for some of the allergies attributed to latex.

Toxicology

Thiram dust is moderately irritating to human skin, eyes, and respiratory mucous membranes. Contact dermatitis has occurred in occupationally exposed workers. A few individuals have experienced sensitization to thiram.[3]

Systemic human poisonings by thiram itself have been very few, probably due to limited absorption in most circumstances involving human exposure. Those which have been reported have been similar clinically to toxic reactions to disulfiram (Antabuse), the ethyl analogue of thiram which has been extensively used in alcohol aversion therapy.[3] In laboratory animals, thiram at high dosage has effects similar to those of disulfiram (hyperactivity, ataxia, loss of muscle tone, dyspnea, and convulsions), but thiram appears to be about 10 times as toxic as disulfiram.

Neither thiram nor disulfiram are cholinesterase inhibitors. Both, however, inhibit the enzyme acetaldehyde dehydrogenase, which is critical to the conversion of acetaldehyde to acetic acid. This is the basis for the "Antabuse reaction" that occurs when ethanol is consumed by a person on regular disulfiram dosage. The reaction includes symptoms of nausea, vomiting, pounding headache, dizziness, faintness, mental confusion, dyspnea, chest and abdominal pain, profuse sweating, and skin rash. In rare instances, Antabuse reactions may have occurred in workers who drank alcohol after previously being exposed to thiram.

Confirmation of Poisoning

Urinary xanthurenic acid excretion has been used to monitor workers exposed to thiram. The test is not generally available.

Treatment: Thiram Toxicosis

1. Skin decontamination. Wash thiram from the skin with soap and water. Flush contamination from the eyes with copious amounts of clean water. If irritation of skin or eyes persists, specialized medical treatment should be obtained.

2. Gastrointestinal decontamination. If a large amount of thiram has been swallowed within 60 minutes of presentation, and effective vomiting has not already occurred, the stomach may be emptied by intubation, aspiration, and lavage, taking all precautions to protect the airway from aspiration of vomitus. Lavage should be followed by instillation of activated charcoal and cathartic. If only a small amount of thiram has been ingested and/or treatment has been delayed, oral administration of activated charcoal and cathartic probably represents optimal management.

3. Intravenous fluids. Appropriate IV fluids should be infused, especially if vomiting and diarrhea are severe. Serum electrolytes and glucose should be monitored and replaced as needed.

Treatment: Acetaldehyde Toxicosis (Antabuse Reaction)

1. Immediate management. Oxygen inhalation, Trendelenburg positioning, and intravenous fluids are usually effective in relieving manifestations of Antabuse reactions.

2. Alochol avoidance. Persons who have absorbed any significant amount of thiocarbamates must avoid alcoholic beverages for at least three weeks. Disposition of thiocarbamates is slow, and their inhibitory effects on enzymes are slowly reversible.

ZIRAM AND FERBAM

These are formulated as flowable and wettable powders, used widely on fruit and nut trees, apples, vegetables, and tobacco.

Toxicology

Dust from these fungicides is irritating to the skin, respiratory tract, and eyes. Prolonged inhalation of ziram is said to have caused neural and visual disturbances, and, in a single case of poisoning, a fatal hemolytic reaction. Theoretically, exposure to ziram or ferbam may predispose the individual to Antabuse reactions if alcohol is ingested after exposure. (See Thiram.) However, no such occurrences have been reported.

Confirmation of Poisoning

No tests for these fungicides or their breakdown products in body fluids are available.

Treatment

1. Skin decontamination. Skin contamination should be washed off with soap and water. Flush contamination from the eyes with copious amounts of water. If dermal or eye irritation persists, specialized medical treatment should be obtained. See Chapter 2.

2. Gastrointestinal decontamination. If substantial amounts of ferbam or ziram have been ingested recently, consideration should be given to gastric emptying. If dosage was small and/or several hours have elapsed since ingestion, oral administration of charcoal and a cathartic probably represents optimal management.

3. Hemolysis. If hemolysis occurs, intravenous fluids should be administered, and induction of diuresis considered.

ETHYLENE BIS DITHIOCARBAMATES (EBDC COMPOUNDS)

MANEB, ZINEB, NABAM, AND MANCOZEB

Maneb and zineb are formulated as wettable and flowable powders. Nabam is provided as a soluble powder and in water solution. Mancozeb is a coordination product of zinc ion and maneb. It is formulated as a dust and as wettable and liquid flowable powders.

Toxicology

These fungicides may cause irritation of the skin, respiratory tract, and eyes. Both maneb and zineb have apparently been responsible for some cases of chronic skin disease in occupationally exposed workers, possibly by sensitization.

Although marked adverse effects may follow injection of EBDC compounds into animals, systemic toxicity by oral and dermal routes is generally low. Nabam exhibits the greatest toxicity, probably due to its greater water solubility and absorbability. Maneb is moderately soluble in water, but mancozeb and zineb are essentially water insoluble. Absorption of the latter fungicides across skin and mucous membranes is probably very limited. Systemic poisonings of humans have been extremely rare. However, zineb apparently precipitated an episode of hemolytic anemia in one worker predisposed by reason of multiple red cell enzyme deficiencies.[4] Maneb exposure has been reported in one person who developed acute renal failure and was treated with hemodialysis.[5] Another person developed behavioral and neurological symptoms including tonic–clonic seizures after handling maneb. He recovered uneventfully with supportive care.[6]

The EBDC compounds are not inhibitors of cholinesterase or of acetaldehyde dehydrogenase. They do not induce cholinergic illness or "Antabuse" reactions.

Confirmation of Poisoining

No tests for these fungicides or their breakdown products in body fluids are available.

Treatment

See Treatment for Substituted Benzenes, p. 139.

THIOPHTHALIMIDES

CAPTAN, CAPTAFOL, AND FOLPET

These agents are widely used to protect seed, field crops, and stored produce. They are formulated as dusts and wettable powders. Captafol is no longer registered for use in the United States.

Toxicology

All of these fungicides are moderately irritating to the skin, eyes, and respiratory tract. Dermal sensitization may occur; captafol appears to have been responsible for several episodes of occupational contact dermatitis.[7,8] No systemic poisonings by thiophthalimides have been reported in humans, although captafol has been reported to have exacerbated asthma after occupational exposure.[9] Laboratory animals given very large doses of captan exhibit hypothermia, irritability, listlessness, anorexia, hyporeflexia, and oliguria, the latter with glycosuria and hematuria.

Confirmation of Poisoning

Captan fungicides are metabolized in the body to yield two metabolites that can be measured in the urine.[10]

Treatment

See Treatment for Substituted Benzenes, p. 139.

COPPER COMPOUNDS

INORGANIC AND ORGANIC COMPOUNDS

Insoluble compounds are formulated as wettable powders and dusts. Soluble salts are prepared as aqueous solutions. Some organometallic compounds are soluble in mineral oils.

A great many commercial copper-containing fungicides are available. Some are mixtures of copper compounds. Others include lime, other metals, and other fungicides. Compositions of specific products can usually be provided by manufacturers or by poison control centers.

Copper-arsenic compounds such as Paris green may still be used in agriculture outside the U.S. Toxicity of these compounds is chiefly due to arsenic content (see Chapter 14, Arsenical Pesticides).

Commercial Products

THIOPHTHALIMIDES

captafol*
  Crisfolatan
  Difolatan
  Foltaf
  Haipen
  Merpafol
  Mycodifol
  Sanspor
captan
  Captaf
  Captanex
  Merpan
  Orthocide
  Vondcaptan
folpet
  Folpan
  Fungitrol II
  Phaltan
  Thiophal

COPPER COMPOUNDS

Inorganic Copper Compounds
copper acetate
copper ammonium carbonate
copper carbonate, basic
copper hydroxide
copper lime dust
copper oxychloride
copper potassium sulfide
copper silicate
copper sulfate
cupric oxide
cuprous oxide
tribasic
  Bordeaux Mixture

Organic Copper Compounds
copper linoleate
copper naphthenate
copper oleate
copper phenyl salicylate
copper quinolinolate
copper resinate

* Discontinued in the U.S.

Toxicology

The dust and powder preparations of copper compounds are irritating to the skin, respiratory tract, and particularly to the eyes. Soluble copper salts (such as the sulfate and acetate) are corrosive to mucous membranes and the cornea. Limited solubility and absorption probably account for the generally low systemic toxicity of most compounds. The more absorbable organic copper compounds exhibit the greatest systemic toxicity in laboratory animals. Irritant effects from occupational exposures to copper-containing fungicides have been fairly frequent. Most of what is known about mammalian toxicity of copper compounds has come from veterinary toxicology (livestock seem uniquely vulnerable) and poisonings in humans due to deliberate ingestion of copper sulfate or to consumption of water or food that had been contained in copper vessels.

Early signs and symptoms of copper poisoning include a metallic taste, nausea, vomiting, and epigastric pain. In more severe poisonings, the gastrointestinal irritation will worsen with hemetemesis and melanotic stools. Jaundice and hepatomegaly are common.[11,12] Hemolysis can occur, resulting in circulatory collapse and shock. Methemoglobinemia has been reported in these cases.[11,13,14] Acute renal failure with oliguria can also occur. Shock is a primary cause of death early in the course, and renal failure and hepatic failure contribute to death more than 24 hours after poisoning.[15]

Treatment

Management of poisonings by ingestion of copper-containing fungicides depends entirely on the chemical nature of the compound: the strongly ionized salts present the greatest hazard; the oxides, hydroxides, oxychloride, and oxysulfate are less likely to cause severe systemic poisoning.

1. Skin decontamination. Dust and powder should be washed from the skin with soap and water. Flush the eyes free of irritating dust, powder, or solution, using clean water or saline. If eye or dermal irritation persists, specialized medical treatment should be obtained. Eye irritation may be severe. See Chapter 2.

2. Anti-corrosive. Give water or milk as soon as possible to dilute the toxicant and mitigate corrosive action on the mouth, esophagus, and gut.

3. Gastrointestinal decontamination. Vomiting is usually spontaneous in acute copper ingestion. Further induction of emesis is contraindicated because the corrosive nature of some copper salts can cause further damage to the esophagus. Further GI decontamination should be determined on a case-by-case basis, as outlined in Chapter 2. Gastric lavage may cause further damage.[15] Charcoal has not been widely studied in metal poisonings as an effective adsorbant.

Caution: Gastric intubation may pose a serious risk of esophageal perforation if corrosive action has been severe. In this event, it may be best to avoid gastric intubation.

4. Intravenous fluids. If indications of systemic illness appear, administer intravenous fluids containing glucose and electrolytes. Monitor fluid balance, and correct blood electrolyte concentrations as needed. If shock develops, give blood transfusions and vasopressor amines, as required.

5. Hemolysis. Monitor plasma for evidence of hemolysis (free hemoglobin) and the red cells for methemoglobin. If hemolysis occurs, alkalinize the urine to about pH 7.5 by adding sodium bicarbonate to the intravenous infusion fluid. Also, mannitol diuresis may be considered. If methemoglobinemia is severe (> 30%), or the patient is cyanotic, administer methylene blue. The dosage for adults/child is 1–2 mg/kg/dose, given as a slow IV push over a few minutes, every 4 hours as needed.[15]

6. Pain management. Severe pain may require the administration of morphine.

7. Chelating agents. The value of chelating agents in copper poisoning has not been established.[16] However, BAL appears to accelerate copper excretion and may alleviate illness. D-penicillamine is the treatment for Wilson's disease due to chronic copper toxicity; however, in the context of severe vomiting and/or mental status changes from an acute ingestion, BAL would be a more likely initial choice.[13,15] For a recommended schedule of dosage for initial therapy with BAL and subsequent penicillamine administration, see Chapter 14, Arsenical Pesticides.

8. Hemodialysis. Although hemodialysis is indicated for patients with renal failure, copper is not effectively removed in the dialysate.[11]

ORGANOMERCURY COMPOUNDS

METHYL MERCURY AND METHOXYETHYL MERCURY COMPOUNDS, PHENYLMERCURIC ACETATE

These fungicides have been formulated as aqueous solutions and dusts. They have been used chiefly as seed protectants. Use of alkyl mercury fungicides in the United States has been virtually prohibited for several years. Phenylmercuric acetate is no longer permitted to be used in the United States.

ORGANOMERCURY COMPOUNDS

Methyl Mercury Compounds
methyl mercury acetate
   propionate
   quinolinolate

Methoxyethyl Mercury Compounds
methoxyethyl mercury acetate
   MEMA
   Panogen
   Panogen M
methoxyethyl mercury chloride
   Ceresan
   Emisan 6
   MEMC

Phenylmercuric Acetate
   Agrosan
   Setrete
   Gallotox
   PMAA
   Shimmer-ex
   Tag HL 331
   Unisan

Toxicology

The mercurial fungicides are among the most toxic pesticides ever developed, for both chronic and acute hazards. Epidemics of severe, often fatal, neurologic disease have occurred when indigent residents of less developed countries consumed methyl mercury-treated grain intended for planting of crops.[17,18] Poisoning has also occurred from eating meat from animals fed mercury-treated seed.[19] Most of what is known of poisoning by organic mercurial fungicides has come from these occurrences.

Organic mercury compounds are efficiently absorbed across the gut and possibly across the skin. Volatile organic mercury is readily taken up across the pulmonary membrane. Methyl mercury is selectively concentrated in the tissue of the nervous system, and also in red blood cells. Other alkyl mercury compounds are probably distributed similarly. Excretion occurs almost entirely by way of the bile into the bowel. The residence half-life of methyl mercury in humans is about 65 days.[20] There is significant conversion of organic mercury to inorganic mercury in the red cell.

Early symptoms of poisoning are metallic taste in the mouth, numbness and tingling of the digits and face, tremor, headache, fatigue, emotional lability, and difficulty thinking. Manifestations of more severe poisoning are incoordination, slurred speech, loss of position sense, hearing loss, constriction of visual fields, spasticity or rigidity of muscle movements, and deterioration of mental capacity. Many poisonings caused by ingestion of organic mercurials have terminated fatally, and a large percentage of survivors have suffered severe permanent neurologic damage.[17-19]

Phenylmercuric acetate is not as extremely toxic as the alkyl mercury compounds. It is not as efficiently absorbed from the gut as methyl mercury.[21] Phenylmercuric acetate had been used to prevent fungal growth in latex paint. There have been reports of acrodynia in persons exposed to mercury vapor from use of interior latex paint. Symptoms include fever, erythema and desquamation of hands and feet, muscular weakness, leg cramps, and personality changes.[22] Phenylmercuric compounds have since been banned from latex paint.[20]

Confirmation of Poisoning

Mercury content of blood and tissues can be measured by atomic absorption spectrometry. Blood levels of 5 mcg/dL or greater are considered elevated for acute exposure.[21] Special procedures are needed for extraction and measurement of organic mercury compounds specifically.

Treatment

Every possible precaution should be taken to avoid exposure to organic mercury compounds. Ingestion of an organic mercury compound, even at low dosage, is life threatening, and management is difficult. Very little can be done to mitigate neurologic damage caused by organic mercurials.

Persons experiencing symptoms (metallic taste in mouth) after inhalation of volatile organic mercury compounds (methyl mercury is the most volatile) should be removed promptly from the contaminated environment and observed closely for indications of neurologic impairment. Following are the basic steps in management of poisoning:

1. Skin decontamination. Skin and hair contaminated by mercury–containing dust or solution should be cleansed with soap and water. Flush contamination from the eyes with clean water. If irritation persists, specialized medical care should be obtained. See Chapter 2.

2. Gastrointestinal decontamination. Consider gastrointestinal decontamination as outlined in Chapter 2.

3. Chelation is an essential part of the management of mercury poisoning. For dosages of specific agents, see Chapter 14, Arsenical Pesticides. Succimer (DMSA) appears to be the most effective agent available in the United States. Dimercaprol (BAL) is contraindicated in these poisonings due to its potential to increase brain levels of mercury.[20] EDTA is apparently of little value in poisonings by organic mercury. D-penicillamine is probably useful, is available in the United States, and has proven effective in reducing the residence half-life of methyl mercury in poisoned humans.[20] 2,3-dimercaptopropane-1-sulfonate acid (DMPS) and N-acetyl-D,L-penicillamine (NAP) are probably also useful but are not currently approved for use in the United States.

4. Hemodialysis. Extracorporeal hemodialysis and hemoperfusion may be considered, although experience to date has not been encouraging.

ORGANOTIN COMPOUNDS

These compounds are formulated as wettable and flowable powders for use mainly as fungicides to control blights on field crops and orchard trees. Fentin chloride was also prepared as an emulsifiable concentrate for use as a molluscicide (Aquatin 20 EC, discontinued 1995). Tributyltin salts are used as fungicides and antifouling agents on ships. They are somewhat more toxic by the oral route than triphenyltin, but toxic actions are otherwise probably similar.

CADMIUM
COMPOUNDS

cadmium chloride*
  Caddy
cadmium succinate*
  Cadminate
cadmium sulfate*
  Cad-Trete
  Crag Turf Fungicide
  Kromad
  Miller 531

* Discontinued in the U.S.

Toxicology

These agents are irritating to the eyes, respiratory tract, and skin. They are probably absorbed to a limited extent by the skin and gastrointestinal tract. Manifestations of toxicity are due principally to effects on the central nervous system: headache, nausea, vomiting, dizziness, and sometimes convulsions and loss of consciousness. Photophobia and mental disturbances occur. Epigastric pain is reported, even in poisoning caused by inhalation. Elevation of blood sugar, sufficient to cause glycosuria, has occurred in some cases. The phenyltin fungicides are less toxic than ethyltin compounds, which have caused cerebral edema, neurologic damage, and death in severely poisoned individuals who were exposed dermally to a medicinal compound of this type.[23] No deaths and very few poisonings have been reported as a result of occupational exposures to phenyltin compounds.

Treatment

1. Skin decontamination. Skin contamination should be removed by washing with soap and water. Flush contaminants from the eyes with clean water or saline. If irritation persists, specialized medical treatment should be obtained. See Chapter 2.

2. Gastrointestinal decontamination. If large amounts of phenyltin compound have been ingested in the past hour, measures may be taken to decontaminate the gastrointestinal tract, as outlined in Chapter 2.

3. Chelating agents. Neither BAL, penicillamine, nor other chelating agents have been effective in lowering tissue stores of organotin compounds in experimental animals.

CADMIUM COMPOUNDS

Cadmium salts have been used to treat fungal diseases affecting turf and the bark of orchard trees. They were formulated as solutions and emulsions. Miller 531 and Crag Turf Fungicide 531 were complexes of cadmium, calcium, copper, chromium, and zinc oxides. They are now marketed as a generic fungicide. Kromad is a mixture of cadmium sebacate, potassium chromate, and thiram. Cad-Trete is a mixture of cadmium chloride and thiram. All cadmium fungicides in the U.S. have been discontinued.

Toxicology

Cadmium salts and oxides are very irritating to the respiratory and gastrointestinal tracts. Inhaled cadmium dust or fumes can cause respiratory toxicity after a latency period of several hours, including a mild, self-limited illness of fever, cough, malaise, headaches, and abdominal pain, similar to metal fume fever. A more severe form of toxicity includes chemical pneumonitis, and is associated with labored breathing, chest pain, and a sometimes fatal hemorrhagic pulmonary edema.[24,25] Symptoms may persist for weeks.

Ingested cadmium causes nausea, vomiting, diarrhea, abdominal pain, and tenesmus. Relatively small inhaled and ingested doses produce serious symptoms. Protracted absorption of cadmium has led to renal damage (proteinuria and azotemia), anemia, liver injury (jaundice), and defective bone structure (pathologic fractures) in chronically exposed persons. Prolonged inhalation of cadmium dust has contributed to chronic obstructive pulmonary disease.[26]

Confirmation of Poisoning

Cadmium can be measured in body fluids by appropriate extraction, followed by flame absorption spectrometry. It is reported that blood cadmium concentrations tend to correlate with acute exposure and urine levels tend to reflect total body burden. Blood levels exceeding 5 mcg/dL suggest excessive exposure.[25] Urinary excretion in excess of 100 mcg per day suggests an unusually high body burden.

Treatment

1. Skin decontamination. Skin contamination should be removed by washing with soap and water. Flush contamination from the eyes with copious amounts of clean water or saline. If irritation persists, specialized medical treatment should be obtained. See Chapter 2.

2. Pulmonary edema. Respiratory irritation resulting from inhalation of small amounts of cadmium dust may resolve spontaneously, requiring no treatment. More severe reactions, including pulmonary edema and pneumonitis, may require aggressive measures, including positive pressure mechanical pulmonary ventilation, monitoring of blood gases, administration of diuretics, steroid medications, and antibiotics.[25] Codeine sulfate may be needed to control cough and chest pain.

3. Gastrointestinal decontamination. The irritant action of ingested cadmium products on the gastrointestinal tract is so strong that spontaneous vomiting and diarrhea often eliminate nearly all unabsorbed cadmium from the gut. If retention of some cadmium in the lower GI tract is suspected, further gastrointestinal decontamination may be considered, as outlined in Chapter 2.

4. Intravenous fluids may be required to overcome dehydration caused by vomiting and diarrhea. Also, fluids limit cadmium toxicity affecting the kidneys and liver. However, great care must be taken to monitor fluid balance and blood electrolyte concentrations, so that failing renal function does not lead to fluid overload.

5. Chelation therapy with calcium disodium EDTA may be considered for acute poisoning, depending on measured cadmium in blood and urine, and the status of renal function. Its therapeutic value in cadmium poisoning has not been established, and use of the agent carries the risk that unduly rapid transfer of cadmium to the kidney may precipitate renal failure. Urine protein and blood urea nitrogen and creatinine should be carefully monitored during therapy. The dosage should be 75 mg/kg/day in three to six divided doses for 5 days. The total dose for the 5-day course should not exceed 500 mg/kg.[27] Succimer (DMSA) has also been used in this poisoning, but has not been demonstrated to be efficacious.

6. Contraindications: Dimercaprol (BAL) is not recommended for treatment of cadmium poisoning, chiefly because of the risk of renal injury by mobilized cadmium.

7. Liver function. Monitor urine content of protein and cells regularly, and perform liver function tests for indications of injury to these organs.

MISCELLANEOUS ORGANIC FUNGICIDES

Some modern organic fungicides are widely used. Reports of adverse effects on humans are few. Some of the known properties of these agents are listed below.

Anilazine is supplied as wettable and flowable powders. Used on vegetables, cereals, coffee, ornamentals, and turf. This product has caused skin irritation in exposed workers. Acute oral and dermal toxicity in laboratory animals is low. Human systemic poisonings have not been reported.

Benomyl is a synthetic organic fungistat having little or no acute toxic effect in mammals. No systemic poisonings have been reported in humans. Although the molecule contains a carbamate grouping, benomyl is not a cholinesterase inhibitor. It is poorly absorbed across skin; whatever is absorbed is promptly metabolized and excreted.

Skin injuries to exposed individuals have occurred, and dermal sensitization has been found among agricultural workers exposed to foliage residues.

Cycloheximide is formulated as wettable powder, sometimes combined with other fungicides. Cycloheximide is a product of fungal culture, effective against fungal diseases of ornamentals and grasses. It is selectively toxic to rats, much less toxic to dogs and monkeys. No human poisonings have been reported. Animals given toxic doses exhibit salivation, bloody diarrhea, tremors, and excitement, leading to coma and death due to cardiovascular collapse. Hydrocortisone increases the rate of survival of deliberately poisoned rats. Atropine, epinephrine, methoxyphenamine, and hexamethonium all relieved the symptoms of poisoning, but did not improve survival.

Dodine is formulated as a wettable powder. It is commonly applied to berries, nuts, peaches, apples, pears, and to trees afflicted with leaf blight. Dodine is a cationic surfactant with antifungal activity. It is absorbed across the skin and is irritating to skin, eyes, and gastrointestinal tract. Acute oral and dermal toxicity in laboratory animals is moderate. Poisonings in humans have not been reported. Based on animal studies, ingestion would probably cause nausea, vomiting, and diarrhea.

Iprodione is supplied as wettable powder and other formulations. It is used on berries, grapes, fruit, vegetables, grasses, and ornamentals, and as a seed dressing. Iprodione exhibits low acute oral and dermal toxicity in laboratory animals. No human poisonings have been reported.

Metalaxyl is supplied as emulsifiable and flowable concentrates. It is used to control soil-borne fungal diseases on fruit trees, cotton, hops, soybeans, peanuts, ornamentals and grasses. Also used as seed dressing. Metalaxyl exhibits low acute oral and dermal toxicity in laboratory animals. No human poisonings have been reported.

Etridiazole is supplied as wettable powder and granules for application to soil as a fungicide and nitrification inhibitor. Contact may result in irritation of skin and eyes. Systemic toxicity is low. Human poisonings have not been reported.

Thiabendazole is widely used as an agricultural fungicide, but most experience with its toxicology in humans has come from medicinal use against intestinal parasites. Oral doses administered for this purpose are far greater than those likely to be absorbed in the course of occupational exposure. Thiabendazole is rapidly metabolized and excreted in the urine, mostly as a conjugated hydroxy-metabolite. Symptoms and signs that sometimes follow ingestion are: dizziness, nausea, vomiting, diarrhea, epigastric distress, lethargy, fever, flushing, chills, rash and local edema, headache, tinnitus, paresthesia, and hypotension. Blood enzyme tests may indicate liver injury. Persons with liver and kidney disease may be unusually vulnerable to toxic effects. Adverse effects from use of thiabendazole as a fungicide have not been reported.

Triadimefon is supplied as wettable powder, emulsifiable concentrate, suspension concentrate, paste, and dry flowable powder. Used on fruit, cereals, vegetables, coffee, ornamentals, sugarcane, pineapple, and turf, triadimefon exhibits moderate acute oral toxicity in laboratory animals, but dermal toxicity is low. It causes irritation if eyes are contaminated. Triadimefon is absorbed across the skin. Overexposures of humans are said to have resulted in hyperactivity followed by sedation.

Triforine is supplied as emulsifiable concentrate and wettable powder. Used on berries, fruit, vegetables, and ornamentals, triforine exhibits low acute oral and dermal toxicity in laboratory animals. Mammals rapidly excrete it chiefly as a urinary metabolite. No human poisonings have been reported.

Confirmation of Poisoining

There are no generally available laboratory tests for these organic fungicides or their metabolites in body fluids.

Treatment

See Treatment for Substituted Benzenes, p. 139.

References

1. Dannaker CJ, Maibach HI, and O'Malley M. Contact urticaria and anaphylaxis to the fungicide chlorothalonil. *Cutis* 1993;52:3120-5.

2. Peters HA, Gocmen A, Cripps DJ, et al. Epidemiology of hexachlorobenzene-induced porphyria in Turkey: Clinical and laboratory follow-up after 25 years. *Arch Neurol* 1992;39:744-9.

3. Dalvi RR. Toxicology of thiram (tetramethylthiuram disulfide): A review. *Vet Hum Toxicol* 1988;30:480-2.

4. Pinkhans J, Djaldetti M, Joshua H, et al. Sulfahemoglobinemia and acute hemolytic anemia with Heinz bodies following contact with a fungicide-zinc ethylene bisdithiocarbamate in a subject with glucose-6-phosphate dehydrogenase deficiency and hypocatalasemia. *Blood* 1963;21:484-93.

5. Koizumi A, Shiojima S, Omiya M, et al. Acute renal failure and maneb (manganouis ethylenebis[dithiocarbamate]) exposure. *JAMA* 1979;242:2583-5.

6. Israeli R, Sculsky M, and Tiberin P. Acute intoxication due to exposure to maneb and zineb: A case with behavioral and central nervous system changes. *Scand J Work Environ Health* 1983;9:47-51.

7. Peluso AM, Tardio M, Adamo F, et al. Multiple sensitization due to bis-dithiocarbamate and thiophthalimide pesticides. *Contact Dermatitis* 1991;25:327.

8. Vilaplana J and Romaguera C. Captan, a rare contact sensitizer in hairdressing. *Contact Dermatitis* 1993;29:107.

9. Royce S, Wald P, Sheppard D, et al. Occupational asthma in a pesticides manufacturing worker. *Chest* 1993;103:295-6.

10. Krieger RI and Thongsinthusak T. Captan metabolism in humans yields two biomarkers, tetrahydrophthalimide (THPI) and thiazolidine-2-thione-4-carboxylic acid (TTCA) in urine. *Drug Chem Toxicol* 1993;16:207-25.

11. Agarwal SK, Tiwari SC, and Dash SC. Spectrum of poisoning requiring haemodialysis in a tertiary care hospital in India. *Int J Artif Organs* 1993;16:20-3.

12. Lamont DL and Duflou JALC. Copper sulfate: Not a harmless chemical. *Am J Forensic Med Pathol* 1988;9:226-7.

13. Chugh KS, Singhal PC, and Sharma BK. Methemoglobinemia in acute copper sulfate poisoning. *Ann Intern Med* 1975;82:226-9.

14. Jantsch W, Kulig K, and Rumack BH. Massive copper sulfate ingestion resulting in hepatotoxicity. *Clin Toxicol* 1984-85;22:585-8.

15. POISINDEX®: Copper poisoning. Englewood, CO: Micromedex, 1998.

16. Hantson P, Lievens M, and Mahieu P. Accidental ingestion of a zinc and copper sulfate preparation. *Clin Toxicol* 1996;34:725-30.

17. Bakir F, Rustam H, Tikritis S, et al. Clinical and epidemiological aspects of methylmercury poisoning. *Postgrad Med J* 1980;56:1-10.

18. Grandjean P, Weihe P, and Nielsen JB. Methylmercury; Significance of intrauterine and postnatal exposures. *Clin Chem* 1994;40:1395-1400.

19. Snyder RD. Congenital mercury poisoning. *New Engl J Med* 1971;284:1014-5.

20. Clarkson TW. Mercury— An element of mystery. *New Engl J Med* 1990;323:1137-8.

21. Agency for Toxic Substances and Disease Registry. Mercury toxicity. *Am Fam Physician* 1992;46:1731-41.

22. Agocs MM, Etzel RA, Parrish RG, et al. Mercury exposure from interior latex paint. *New Engl J Med* 1990;323:1096-100.

23. Colosio C, Tomasini M, Cairoli S, et al. Occupational triphenyltin acetate poisoning: A case report. *Br J Ind Med* 1991;48:136-9.

24. Barnhart S and Rosenstock L. Cadmium chemical pneumonitis. *Chest* 1984;86:789-91.

25. Ando Y, Shibata E, Tsuchiyama F, et al. Elevated urinary cadmium concentrations in a patient with acute cadmium pneumonitis. *Scand J Work Environ Health* 1996;22:150-3.

26. Hendrick DJ. Occupational and chronic obstructive pulmonary disease (COPD). *Thorax* 1996;51:947-55.

27. Klaassen CD. Heavy metals and heavy metal antagonists. In: Gilman AG, Rall TW, Niew AS, et al (eds). Goodman and Gilman's The Pharmacological Basis of Therapeutics, 3rd ed. New York: Pergamon Press, 1990, pp. 1605-6.

Fumigants

Fumigants have remarkable capacities for diffusion, a property essential to their function. Some readily penetrate rubber and neoprene personal protective gear, as well as human skin. They are rapidly absorbed across the pulmonary membrane, gut, and skin. Special adsorbents are required in respirator canisters to protect exposed workers from airborne fumigant gases. Even these may not provide complete protection when air concentrations of fumigants are high.

The packaging and formulation of fumigants are complex. Fumigants which are gases at room temperature (methyl bromide, ethylene oxide, sulfur dioxide, hydrogen cyanide, sulfuryl fluoride) are provided in compressed gas cylinders. Liquids are marketed in cans or drums. Solids which sublime, such as naphthalene, must be packaged so as to prevent significant contact with air before they are used.

Mixtures of fumigants have several advantages. Carbon tetrachloride reduces the explosiveness of carbon disulfide and acrylonitrile. Chloropicrin, having a strong odor and irritant effect, is often added as a "warning agent" to other liquid fumigants.

Liquid halocarbons and carbon disulfide evaporate into the air while naphthalene sublimes. Paraformaldehyde slowly depolymerizes to formaldehyde. Aluminum phosphide slowly reacts with water vapor in the air to liberate phosphine, an extremely toxic gas. Metam sodium, also a fumigant, is covered under thiocarbamates in Chapter 15, Fungicides.

Toxicology *(in alphabetical order)*

Acrolein (acrylaldehyde) is an extremely irritating gas used as a fumigant and an aquatic herbicide. The vapor causes lacrimation and upper respiratory tract irritation, which may lead to laryngeal edema, bronchospasm, and delayed pulmonary edema. The consequences of ingestion are essentially the same as those that follow ingestion of formaldehyde. Contact with the skin may cause blistering.

Acrylonitrile is biotransformed in the body to hydrogen cyanide. Toxicity and mechanisms of poisoning are essentially the same as for cyanide (see under hydrogen cyanide below), except that acrylonitrile is irritating to the eyes and to the upper respiratory tract.

Carbon disulfide vapor is only moderately irritating to upper respiratory membranes, but it has an offensive "rotten cabbage" odor. Acute toxicity is due chiefly to effects on the central nervous system. Inhalation of high concentrations for short periods has caused headache, dizziness, nausea, hallucinations, delirium, progressive paralysis, and death from respiratory failure. More prolonged exposure to lesser amounts has lead to blindness, deafness, paresthesia, painful neuropathy, and paralysis. Carbon disulfide is a potent skin irritant, often causing severe burns. Long-term occupational exposures have been shown to accelerate atherosclerosis, leading to ischemic myocardiopathy, polyneuropathy, and gastrointestinal dysfunction.[1] Toxic damage to the liver and kidneys may result in severe functional deficits of these organs. Reproductive failure has been noted.

Carbon tetrachloride is less toxic than chloroform as a central nervous system depressant, but is much more severely hepatotoxic, particularly following ingestion. Liver cell damage is apparently due to free radicals generated in the process of initial dechlorination.[2] Cardiac arrhythmias, progressing to fibrillation, may follow inhalation of high concentrations of carbon tetrachloride or ingestion of the liquid. Kidney injury also occurs sometimes with minimal hepatic toxicity. The kidney injury may be manifested by acute tubular necrosis or by azotemia and general renal failure. Even topical exposure has resulted in acute renal toxicity.[3]

Chloroform has an agreeable sweet odor and is only slightly irritating to the respiratory tract. It is well absorbed from the lungs and is also absorbed from the skin and gastrointestinal tract. It is a powerful central nervous system depressant (in fact, an anesthetic).[4] Inhalation of toxic concentrations in air leads to dizziness, loss of sensation and motor power, and then unconsciousness. Inhalation of large amounts causes cardiac arrhythmias, sometimes progressing to ventricular fibrillation. Large absorbed doses damage the functional cells of the liver and kidney. Ingestion is more likely to cause serious liver and kidney injury than is inhalation of the vapor.

Chloropicrin is severely irritating to the upper respiratory tract, eyes, and skin. Inhalation of an irritant concentration sometimes leads to vomiting. Ingestion could be expected to cause a corrosive gastroenteritis.

Dibromochloropropane is irritating to skin, eyes, and the respiratory tract. Eye damage has resulted from repeated exposure to the vapors. When absorbed, it causes headache, nausea, vomiting, ataxia, and slurred speech. Liver and kidney damage are prominent features of acute poisoning. Chronic exposure to relatively low concentrations has led to temporary or permanent sterility of workers in a manufacturing plant, by causing diffuse necrosis of seminiferous tubule cells. Because it is much less odiferous than ethylene dibromide, exposure of workers to toxic concentrations of DBCP is more likely. Its use has been cancelled in the U.S.

Dichloropropene and dichloropropane are strongly irritating to the skin, eyes, and respiratory tract. Bronchospasm may result from inhalation of high concentrations. Liver, kidney, and cardiac toxicity are seen in animals, but there are limited data in humans. It appears that risk of such toxicity is relatively low for humans except via ingestion of large quantities.

Commercial Products

HALOCARBONS

carbon tetrachloride*
chloroform*
   trichloromethane
chloropicrin
   Aquinite
   Dojyopicrin
   Dolochlor
   Larvacide
   Pic-Clor
dibromochloropropane*
   Nemafume
   Nemanax
   Nemaset
1,2-dichloropropane*
   propylene dichloride
1,3-dichloropropene
   D-D92
   Telone II Soil Fumigant
ethylene dibromide*
   Bromofume
   Celmide
   dibromoethane
   E-D-Bee
   EDB
   Kopfume
   Nephis
ethylene dichloride*
   dichloroethane
   EDC
methyl bromide
   Celfume
   Kayafume
   Meth-O-Gas
   MeBr
   Sobrom 98
methylene chloride*
paradichlorobenzene

HYDROCARBONS

naphthalene

NITROGEN COMPOUNDS

acrylonitrile*
hydrogen cyanide*
   hydrocyanic acid
   prussic acid

(Continued on the next page)

OXIDES AND ALDEHYDES

acrolein
    Magnacide B
    Magnacide H
1,2-epoxyethane
ethylene oxide
    ETO
formaldehyde
oxirane
paraformaldehyde

PHOSPHORUS COMPOUNDS

phosphine (liberated from
aluminum phosphide or
magnesium phosphide)
    Agtoxin
    Alphos
    Fumex
    Fumitoxin
    Phostoxin
    Quickfos
    Sanifume
    Shaphos
    others

SULFUR COMPOUNDS

carbon disulfide*
sulfur dioxide
sulfuryl fluoride
    Vikane

* Discontinued in the U.S.

Ethylene dibromide is a severe irritant to skin, eyes, and respiratory tract. The liquid causes blistering and erosion of skin, and is corrosive to the eyes. Once absorbed, it may cause pulmonary edema and central nervous system depression. Damage to testicular tissue has occurred in animals.[5] Long-term exposure may have some damaging effect on testicular tissue. Persons poisoned by ingestion have suffered chemical gastroenteritis, liver necrosis, and renal tubular damage. Death is usually due to respiratory or circulatory failure. A powerful disagreeable odor is advantageous in warning occupationally exposed workers of the presence of this gas.

Ethylene dichloride is moderately irritating to the eyes and respiratory tract. Respiratory symptoms may have a delayed onset. It depresses the central nervous system, induces cardiac arrhythmias, and damages the liver and kidney, in much the same way as carbon tetrachloride. Symptoms and signs of poisoning include headache, nausea, vomiting, dizziness, diarrhea, hypotension, cyanosis, and unconsciousness.

Ethylene oxide and propylene oxide are irritants to all tissues they contact. Aqueous solutions of ethylene oxide cause blistering and erosion of the affected skin. The area of skin may thereafter be sensitized to the fumigant. Inhalation of high concentrations is likely to cause pulmonary edema and cardiac arrhythmias. Headache, nausea, vomiting, weakness, and a persistent cough are common early manifestations of acute poisoning. Coughing of bloody, frothy sputum is characteristic of pulmonary edema.

Airborne **formaldehyde** is irritating to the eyes and to membranes of the upper respiratory tract. In some individuals, it is a potent sensitizer, causing allergic dermatitis. In addition, it has been associated with asthma-like symptoms, though there remains some controversy as to whether these represent true allergic asthma caused by formaldehyde.[6,7,8] High air concentrations may cause laryngeal edema, asthma, or tracheobronchitis, but apparently not pulmonary edema. Aqueous solutions in contact with the skin cause hardening and roughness, due to superficial coagulation of the keratin layer. Ingested formaldehyde attacks the membrane lining of the stomach and intestine, causing necrosis and ulceration. Absorbed formaldehyde is rapidly converted to formic acid. The latter is partly responsible for the metabolic acidosis that is characteristic of formaldehyde poisoning. Circulatory collapse and renal failure may follow the devastating effects of ingested formaldehyde on the gut, leading to death. Paraformaldehyde is a polymer which slowly releases formaldehyde into the air. Toxicity is somewhat less than that of formaldehyde, because of the slow evolution of gas.

Hydrogen cyanide gas causes poisoning by inactivating cytochrome oxidase, the final enzyme essential to mammalian cellular respiration. The patient will have signs of severe hypoxia, however, and in some cases may not appear cyanotic. This is due to the failure of hemoglobin reduction in the face of loss of cellular respiration. This will result in a pink or red color to the skin and arteriolization of retinal veins. In addition to the suggestive physical findings, one may also find an unusually high pO_2 on a venous blood gas.[9] Cyanosis is a late sign and indicates circulatory collapse.

The cells of the brain appear to be the most vulnerable to cyanide action. Presenting signs are nonspecific and can be found with many poisonings. Unconsciousness and death may occur immediately following inhalation of a high cyanide concentration, respiratory failure being the principal mechanism. Metabolic acidosis is another common presenting sign. Lesser exposures cause a constriction and numbness in the throat, stiffness of the jaw, salivation, nausea, vomiting, lightheadedness, and apprehension. Worsening of the poisoning is manifest as violent tonic or clonic convulsions. Fixed, dilated pupils, bradycardia, and irregular gasping respiration (or apnea) are typical of profound poisoning. The heart often continues to beat after breathing has stopped.[9,10] A bitter almond odor to the breath or vomitus may be a clue to poisoning, but not all individuals are able to detect this odor.[9]

Methyl bromide is colorless and nearly odorless, but is severely irritating to the lower respiratory tract, sometimes inducing pulmonary edema, hemorrhage, or a confluent pneumonia. The onset of respiratory distress may be delayed 4–12 hours after exposure. It is a central nervous system depressant, but may also cause convulsions. Early symptoms of acute poisoning include headache, dizziness, nausea, vomiting, tremor, slurred speech, and ataxia. The more severe cases of poisoning exhibit myoclonic and generalized tonic clonic seizures, which are sometimes refractory to initial therapy. Residual neurological deficits including myoclonic seizures, ataxia, muscle weakness, tremors, behavioral disturbances, and diminished reflexes may persist in more severely poisoned patients.[11,12] If liquid methyl bromide contacts the skin, severe burning, itching, and blister formation occur. Skin necrosis may be deep and extensive.

Methylene chloride is one of the less toxic halocarbons. It is absorbed by inhalation and to a limited extent across the skin. Exposure to high concentrations may cause central nervous system depression, manifested as fatigue, weakness, and drowsiness. Some absorbed methylene chloride is degraded to carbon monoxide in humans, yielding increased blood concentrations of carboxyhemoglobin. However, concentrations are rarely high enough to cause symptoms of carbon monoxide poisoning. Ingestion has caused death from gastrointestinal hemorrhage, severe liver damage, coma, shock, metabolic acidosis, and renal injury. In laboratory animals, extraordinary dosage has caused irritability, tremor, and narcosis, leading to death. When heated to that point of decomposition, one of the products is the highly toxic phosgene gas that has caused a significant acute pneumonitis.[13]

Naphthalene is a solid white hydrocarbon long used in ball, flake, or cake form as a moth repellent. It sublimes slowly. The vapor has a sharp, pungent odor that is irritating to the eyes and upper respiratory tract. Inhalation of high concentrations causes headache, dizziness, nausea, and vomiting. Intensive prolonged inhalation exposure, or ingestion or dermal exposure (from contact with heavily treated fabric) may cause hemolysis, particularly in persons afflicted with glucose-6-phosphate dehydrogenase deficiency.[14] The inheritance of glucose-6-phosphate dehydrogenase (G-6-PD) deficiency is by a sex-linked gene with intermediate dominance. For this reason it is most commonly expressed in heterozygous males. However, homozygous females, who are far less common, will have a similar expression. Heterozygous females have only a mild depression of this enzyme. This illness is most common in non-white African and African-American ethnic groups. It is also seen in some Mediterranean ethnic populations.

It is actually the metabolites of naphthalene that are responsible for the hemolysis.[15] Secondary renal tubular damage may ensue from the naphthol and from the products of hemolysis. Convulsions and coma may occur, particularly in children. In infants, high levels of hemoglobin, methemoglobin, and bilirubin in the plasma may lead to encephalopathy. Kernicterus has been specifically described as a complication of exposure to naphthalene with severe hemolysis and resulting hyperbilirubinemia. Some individuals exhibit dermal sensitivity to naphthalene.

Paradichlorobenzene is solid at room temperature, and is now widely used as a moth repellent, air freshener, and deodorizer in homes and in public facilities. The vapor is only mildly irritating to the nose and eyes. Liver injury and tremor may occur following ingestion of large amounts. Although accidental ingestions, especially by children, have been fairly common, symptomatic human poisonings have been rare. Other stereoisomers of dichlorobenzene are more toxic than the para-isomer.

Phosphine gas is extremely irritating to the respiratory tract. It also produces severe systemic toxicity. It is used as a fumigant by placing solid aluminum phosphide (phostoxin) near produce or in other storage spaces. Through hydrolysis, phosphine gas is slowly released. Most severe acute exposures have involved ingestion of the solid aluminum phosphide, which is rapidly converted to phosphine by acid hydrolysis in the stomach. Poisoning due to ingestion carries a high mortality rate (50 to 90%).[16,17] Mechanisms of toxicity are not well understood. Extracellular magnesium levels have been found to be slightly elevated, suggesting a depletion of intracellular magnesium from myocardial damage.[18]

Poisonings had become quite frequent during the late 1980s and early 1990s in some parts of India.[16,17] The principal manifestations of poisoning are fatigue, nausea, headache, dizziness, thirst, cough, shortness of breath, tachycardia, chest tightness, paresthesia, and jaundice. Cardiogenic shock is present in more severe cases. Pulmonary edema is a common cause of death. In other fatalities, ventricular arrythmias, conduction disturbances, and asystole developed.[16,19] Odor is said to resemble that of decaying fish.

Sulfur dioxide is a highly irritant gas, so disagreeable that persons inhaling it are usually prompted to seek uncontaminated air as soon as possible. However, laryngospasm and pulmonary edema have occurred, occasionally leading to severe respiratory distress and death. It is sometimes a cause of reactive airways disease in occupationally exposed persons.

Sulfuryl fluoride has been used extensively for structural fumigation. Although use experience has generally been good, some fatalities have occurred when fumigated buildings have been prematurely reentered by unprotected individuals.[20] Since this material is heavier than air, fatal hypoxia may follow early reentry. Manifestations of poisoning have been nose, eye, and throat irritation, weakness, nausea, vomiting, dyspnea, cough, restlessness, muscle twitching, and seizures. Renal injury may induce proteinuria and azotemia.

Confirmation of Poisoning

There are no practical tests for absorbed **alkyl oxides, aldehydes,** or **phosphine** that would be helpful in diagnosis of poisoning.

Carbon disulfide can be measured in urine by gas chromatography, but the test is not generally available.

Cyanide ion from **cyanide** itself or **acrylonitrile** can be measured in whole blood and urine by an ion-specific electrode or by colorimetry. Symptoms of toxicity may appear at blood levels above 0.10 mg per liter.[10] Urine cyanide is usually less than 0.30 mg per liter in nonsmokers, but as much as 0.80 mg per liter in smokers. Thiocyanate, the metabolite of cyanide, can also be measured in blood and urine. It is elevated at blood levels exceeding 12 mg per liter.[10] Urine thiocyanate is usually less than 4 mg per liter in nonsmokers, but may be as high as 17 mg per liter in smokers.

Methyl bromide yields inorganic bromide in the body. Methyl bromide itself has a short half-life and is usually not detectable after 24 hours. The bromide anion is slowly excreted in the urine (half-life about 10 days), and is the preferred method of serum measurement.[11] The serum from persons having no exceptional exposure to bromide usually contains less than 1 mg bromide ion per 100 mL. The possible contributions of medicinal bromides to elevated blood content and urinary excretion must be considered, but if methyl bromide is the exclusive source, serum bromide exceeding 6 mg per 100 mL probably means some absorption, and 15 mg per 100 mL is consistent with symptoms of acute poisoning. Inorganic bromide is considerably less toxic than methyl bromide; serum concentrations in excess of 150 mg per 100 mL occur commonly in persons taking inorganic bromide medications. In some European countries, blood bromide concentrations are monitored routinely in workers exposed to methyl bromide. Blood levels over 3 mg per 100 mL are considered a warning that personal protective measures must be improved. A bromide concentration over 5 mg per 100 mL requires that the worker be removed from the fumigant-contaminated environment until blood concentrations decline to less than 3 mg per 100 mL.

Methylene chloride is converted to carbon monoxide in the body, generating carboxyhemoglobinemia, which can be measured by clinical laboratories.

Naphthalene is converted mainly to alpha naphthol in the body and promptly excreted in conjugated form in the urine. Alpha naphthol can be measured by gas chromatography. Many halocarbons can be measured in blood by gas chromatographic methods. Some can be measured in the expired air as well.

Paradichlorobenzene is metabolized mainly to 2,5-dichlorophenol, which is conjugated and excreted in the urine. This product can be measured chromatographically.

A serum fluoride concentration of 0.5 mg per liter was measured in one fatality from **sulfuryl fluoride** fumigation. Serum fluoride in persons not exceptionally exposed rarely exceeds 0.1 mg per liter.

Large industrial concerns sometimes monitor human absorption of halocarbons by analysis of expired air. Similar technology is available in some departments of anesthesiology. These analyses are rarely needed to identify the offending toxicant, because this is known from the exposure history. In managing difficult cases of poisoning, however, it may be helpful to monitor breath concentrations of toxic gas to evaluate disposition of the fumigant. Testing of the urine for protein and red cells is needed to detect renal injury. Free hemoglobin in urine most likely reflects hemolysis, as from naphthalene. Elevations of alkaline phosphatase, lactate dehydrogenase (LDH), serum GGT, ALT, AST, and certain other enzymes are sensitive indices of insult to liver cells. More severe damage increases plasma concentrations of bilirubin. The chest x-ray may be used to confirm the occurrence of pulmonary edema. Electromyography may be useful in evaluating peripheral nerve injury. Sperm counts may be appropriate for workers exposed to **dibromochloropropane** and **ethylene dibromide**.

Some occupational health agencies now urge periodic neurologic and neuropsychologic testing of workers heavily exposed to fumigants and solvents to detect injury to the nervous system as early as possible. This would be particularly desirable in the case of exposures to such agents as methyl bromide and carbon disulfide which have well-documented chronic neurotoxic effects.

Treatment

1. Skin decontamination. Flush contaminating fumigants from the skin and eyes with copious amounts of water or saline for at least 15 minutes. Some fumigants are corrosive to the cornea and may cause blindness. Specialized medical treatment should be obtained promptly following decontamination. Skin contamination may cause blistering and deep chemical burns. Absorption of some fumigants across the skin may be sufficient to cause systemic poisoning in the absence of fumigant inhalation. For all these reasons, decontamination of eyes and skin must be immediate and thorough. See Chapter 2.

2. Physical placement. Remove victims of fumigant inhalation to fresh air immediately. Even though initial symptoms and signs are mild, keep the victim quiet, in a semi-reclining position. Minimum physical activity limits the likelihood of pulmonary edema.

3. Respiration. If victim is not breathing, clear the airway of secretions and resuscitate with positive pressure oxygen apparatus. If this is not available, use chest compression to sustain respiration. If victim is pulseless, employ cardiac resuscitation.

4. Pulmonary edema. If pulmonary edema is evident, there are several measures available to sustain life. Medical judgment must be relied upon, however, in the management of each case. The following procedures are generally recommended:

- Put the victim in a sitting position with a backrest.

- Use intermittent and/or continuous positive pressure oxygen to relieve hypoxemia. (Do not give oxygen at greater concentrations or longer periods than necessary, because it may exaggerate the fumigant injury to lung tissue. Monitor arterial pO_2.)

- Slowly administer furosemide, 40 mg, intravenously (0.5-1 mg/kg in children up to 20 mg), to reduce venous load by inducing diuresis. Consult package insert for additional directions and warnings.

Some patients may benefit from careful administration of anxiolytic drugs. Whenever possible, such patients should be managed by intensivists in an intensive care center. Limit victim's physical activity for at least 4 weeks. Severe physical weakness usually indicates persistent pulmonary injury. Serial pulmonary function testing may be useful in assessing recovery.

5. Shock. Combat shock by placing victim in the Trendelenburg position and administering plasma, whole blood, and/or electrolyte and glucose solutions intravenously, with great care, to avoid pulmonary edema. Central venous pressure should be monitored continuously. Vasopressor amines must be given with great caution, because of the irritability of the myocardium.

6. Control convulsions. Seizures are most likely to occur in poisonings by methyl bromide, hydrogen cyanide, acrylonitrile, phosphine, and carbon disulfide. See Chapter 2 for seizure management. In some cases of methyl bromide, seizures have been refractory to benzodiazepines and diphenylhydantoin, and the authors resorted to anesthesia using thiopental.[11]

7. Gastrointestinal decontamination. If a fumigant liquid or solid has been ingested less than an hour prior to treatment, consider gastric emptying, followed by activated charcoal, as suggested in Chapter 2.

8. Fluid balance should be monitored, and urine sediment should be checked regularly for indications of tubular injury. Measure serum alkaline phosphatase, LDH, ALT, AST, and bilirubin to assess liver injury.

9. Extracorporeal hemodialysis may be needed to regulate extracellular fluid composition if renal failure supervenes. It is probably not very effective in removing lipophilic fumigant compounds from blood, but it is, of course, effective in controlling extracellular fluid composition if renal failure occurs.

10. Specific fumigants. Certain specific measures are recommended in poisonings by particular fumigants (carbon disulfide, carbon tetrachloride, naphthalene, phosphine gas, and hydrogen cyanide and acrylonitrile):

- **Carbon Disulfide**: Mild poisonings by carbon disulfide inhalation may be managed best by no more than careful observation, even though sensory hallucinations, delirium, and behavioral aberrations can be alarming. Severe poisonings may require specific measures. If manic behavior threatens the safety of the victim, diazepam (5-10 mg in adults, 0.2-0.4 mg/kg in children), administered slowly, intravenously, may be helpful as a tranquilizer. Give as much as is necessary to achieve sedation. Do not give catecholamine-releasing agents such as reserpine and amphetamines.

- **Carbon Tetrachloride**: For carbon tetrachloride poisoning, several treatment measures have been suggested to limit the severity of hepatic necrosis. Hyperbaric oxygen has been used with some success.[2] Oral administration of N-acetyl cysteine (Mucomyst[R]) may be worthwhile as a means of reducing free radical injury.[21] Dilute the proprietary 20% product 1:4 in a carbonated beverage, and give about 140 mg/kg body weight of the diluted solution as a loading dose. Then give 70 mg/kg every 4 hours after the loading dose for a total of 17 doses. (This dosage schedule is used for acetaminophen poisonings.) Administration via duodenal tube may be necessary in a few patients who cannot tolerate Mucomyst.[22] Intravenous administration of N-acetyl cysteine may be used; more information is available through poison control centers.

- **Naphthalene**: Naphthalene toxicosis caused by vapor inhalation can usually be managed simply by removing the individual to fresh air. Skin contamination should be removed promptly by washing with soap and water. Eye contamination should be removed by flushing with copious amounts of clean water. Eye irritation may be severe, and if it persists, should receive ophthalmalogic attention.

  Examine the plasma for evidence of hemolysis: a reddish-brown tinge, especially in the blood smear for "ghosts" and Heinz bodies. If present, monitor red blood cell count and hematocrit for anemia, urine for protein and cells. Measure direct-and indirect-reacting bilirubin in the plasma. Monitor fluid balance and blood electrolytes. If possible, monitor urinary excretion of naphthol to assess severity of poisoning and clinical progress.

If hemolysis is clinically significant, administer intravenous fluids to accelerate urinary excretion of the naphthol metabolite and protect the kidney from products of hemolysis. Use Ringer's lactate or sodium bicarbonate to keep urine pH above 7.5. Consider the use of mannitol or furosemide to promote diuresis. If urine flow declines, intravenous infusions must be stopped to prevent fluid overload and hemodialysis should be considered.[15] If anemia is severe, blood transfusions may be needed.

- **Phosphine Gas:** Recent experience in India suggests that therapy with magnesium sulfate may decrease the likelihood of a fatal outcome.[16,19,23] The mechanism is unclear, but may possibly be due to the membrane stabilization properties of magnesium in protecting the heart from fatal arrythmias. In one series of 90 patients, magnesium sulfate was found to decrease the mortality from 90% to 52%.[16] Two controlled studies have been done, one of which showed a reduction in mortality from 52% to 22%.[23] The other study found no effect on mortality.[24] The dosage for magnesium sulfate is: 3 grams during the first 3 hours as a continous infusion, followed by 6 grams per 24 hours for the next 3 to 5 days.[16]

- **Hydrogen Cyanide and Acrylonitrile**: Poisonings by hydrogen cyanide and acrylonitrile gases or liquids are treated essentially the same as poisoning by cyanide salts. Because cyanide is so promptly absorbed following ingestion, treatment should commence with prompt administration of oxygen and antidotes. Gastrointestinal decontamination should be considered if the patient presents within a short interval after ingestion, and **only** after the above life-saving treatment has commenced. Ipecac should be avoided due to the potential for rapid onset of loss of consciousness.

The three antidotes — amyl nitrite, sodium nitrite, and sodium thiosulfate — are available as a kit called the Lilly Cyanide Antidote Kit, available from Eli Lilly and Company, Indianapolis, IN. The dosages vary between adults and children and are outlined below.

Dosage of Cyanide Antidotes

Adults:

- Administer **oxygen** continuously. Hyperbaric oxygen has been evaluated as effective in this condition.[25] If respiration fails, maintain pulmonary ventilation mechanically.

- Administer **amyl nitrite** ampules by inhalation for 15–30 seconds of every minute, while a fresh solution of 3% sodium nitrite is being prepared. This solution is ready prepared in commercial cyanide antidote kits.

- As soon as solution is available, inject intravenously 10 mL of 3% **sodium nitrite** solution over a 5-minute interval, keeping the needle in place.

Caution: Monitor pulse and blood pressure during administration of amyl nitrite and sodium nitrite. If systolic blood pressure falls below 80 mm Hg, slow or stop nitrite administration until blood pressure recovers.

- Follow sodium nitrite injection with an infusion of 50 mL of 25% aqueous solution of **sodium thiosulfate** administered over a 10-minute period. Initial adult dose should not exceed 12.5 g.

- If symptoms persist or recur, treatment by sodium nitrite and sodium thiosulfate should be repeated at half the dosages listed above.

- Measure hemoglobin and methemoglobin in blood. If more than 50% of total hemoglobin has been converted to methemoglobin, blood transfusion or exchange transfusion should be considered, because conversion back to normal hemoglobin proceeds slowly.

Children:

- Give amyl nitrite, oxygen, and mechanical respiratory support as recommended for adults. The following dosages of antidotes have been recommended for children.[26]

- Children over 25 kg body weight should receive adult dosages of sodium nitrite and sodium thiosulfate.

- Children less than 25 kg body weight should first have two 3–4 mL samples of blood drawn and then, through the same needle, receive 0.15–0.33 mL/kg up to 10 mL of the 3% solution of sodium nitrite injected over a 5-minute interval. Following sodium nitrite, administer an infusion of 1.65 mL/kg of 25% sodium thiosulfate at a rate of 3–5 mL per minute.

... continued

- At this point, determine the hemoglobin content of the pretreatment blood sample. If symptoms and signs of poisoning persist or return, give supplemental infusions of sodium nitrite and sodium thiosulfate based on hemoglobin level, as presented in the table. These recommended quantities are calculated to avoid life-threatening methemoglobinemia in anemic children. They are aimed at converting approximately 40% of circulating hemoglobin to methemoglobin. If possible, monitor blood methemoglobin concentrations as treatment proceeds.

RECOMMENDED DOSAGES OF SUPPLEMENTAL SODIUM NITRITE AND SODIUM THIOSULFATE BASED ON HEMOGLOBIN LEVEL

Initial Hemoglobin Concentration g/100 mL	Volume of 3% Sodium Nitrite mL/kg	Dose 25% Sodium Thiosulfate mL/kg
14.0	0.20	1.00
12.0	0.16	0.83
10.0	0.14	0.68
8.0	0.11	0.55

Although various cobalt salts, chelates, and organic combinations have shown some promise as antidotes to cyanide, they are not generally available in the United States. None has been shown to surpass the nitrite–thiosulfate regimen in effectiveness.

References

1. Wilcosky TC and Tyroler HA. Mortality from heart disease among workers exposed to solvents. *J Occup Med* 1983;25:879-85.

2. Truss C and Killenberg P. Treatment of carbon tetrachloride poisoning with hyperbaric oxygen. *Gastroenterology* 1982;82:767-9.

3. Perez AJ, Courel M, Sobrado J, et al. Acute renal failure after topical application of carbon tetrachloride. *Lancet* 1987;1:515-6.

4. Dykes MH. Halogenated hydrocarbon ingestion. *Intern Anesthesiol Clin* 1970;8:357-68.

5. Amir D. The spermicidal effect of ethylene dibromide in bulls and rams. *Mol Reprod Dev* 1991;28:99-109.

6. Smedley J. Is formaldehyde an important cause of allergic respiratory disease? *Clin Exp Allergy* 1996;26:247-9.

7. Krzyzanowski M, Quackenboss JJ, and Lebowitz MD. Chronic respiratory effects of indoor formaldehyde exposure. *Environ Res* 1990;52:117-25.

8. Harving H, Korsgaard J, Pedersen OF, et al. Pulmonary function and bronchial reactivity in asthmatics during low-level formaldehyde exposure. *Lung* 1990;168:15-21.

9. Johnson RP and Mellors JW. Arteriolization of venous blood gases: A clue to the diagnosis of cyanide poisoning. *J Emerg Med* 1988;6:401-4.

10. Yen D, Tsai J, Wang LM, et al. The clinical experience of acute cyanide poisoning. *Am J Emerg Med* 1995;13:524-8.

11. Hustinx WNM, van de Laar RTH, van Huffelen A, et al. Systemic effects of inhalational methyl bromide poisoning: A study of nine cases occupationally exposed due to inadvertent spread during fumigation. *Br J Ind Med* 1993;50:155-9.

12. Deschamps FJ and Turpin JC. Methyl bromide intoxication during grain store fumigation. *Occupat Med* 1996;48:89-90.

13. Snyder RW, Mishel HS, and Christensen GC. Pulmonary toxicity following exposure to methylene chloride and its combustion product, phosgene. *Chest* 1992;101:860-1.

14. Shannon K and Buchanan GR. Severe hemolytic anemia in black children with glucose-6-phosphate dehydrogenase deficiency. *Pediatrics* 1982;70:364-9.

15. Gosselin RE, Smith HC, and Hodge HC (eds). Naphthalene. In: Clinical Toxicology of Commercial Products, 5th ed. Baltimore: Williams & Wilkins, 1984, pp. III-307-11.

16. Katira R, Elhence GP, Mehrotra ML, et al. A study of aluminum phosphide poisoning with special reference to electrocardiographic changes. *J Assoc Physicians India* 1990;38:471-3.

17. Singh S, Singh D, Wig N, et al. Aluminum phosphide ingestion: A clinico-pathologic study. *Clin Toxicol* 1996;34:703-6.

18. Singh RB, Singh RG, and Singh U. Hypermagnesemia following aluminum phosphide poisoning. *Int J Clin Pharmacol Ther Toxicol* 1991;29:82-5.

19. Gupta S and Ahlawat SK. Aluminum phosphide poisoning: A review. *Clin Toxicol* 1995;33:19-24.

20. Scheuerman EH. Suicide by exposure to sulfuryl fluoride. *J Forensic Sci* 1986;31:1154-8.

21. Ruprah M, Mant TGK, and Flanagan RJ. Acute carbon tetrachloride poisoning in 19 patients: Implications for diagnosis and treatment. *Lancet* 1985;1:1027-9.

22. Anker AL and Smilkenstein MJ. Acetaminophen: Concepts and controversies. *Emerg Med Clin North Am* 1994;12:335-49.

23. Chugh SN, Kumar P, Sharma A, et al. Magnesium status and parenteral magnesium sulphate therapy in acute aluminum phosphide intoxication. *Magnesium Res* 1994;7:289-94.

24. Siwach SB, Singh P, Ahlawat S, et al. Serum and tissue magnesium content in patients of aluminum phosphide poisoning and critical evaluation of high dose magnesium sulphate therapy in reducing mortality. *J Assoc Physicians India* 1994;42:107-10.

25. Myers RAM and Schnitzer BM. Hyperbaric oxygen use: Update 1984. *Postgrad Med* 1984;76:83-95.

26. Mofenson HC, Greensher J, Horowitz R, and Berlin CM. Treatment of cyanide poisoning. *Pediatrics* 1970;46:793-6.

CHAPTER 17

Rodenticides

A wide variety of materials are used as rodenticides. They pose particular risks for accidental poisonings for several reasons. First, as agents specifically designed to kill mammals, often their toxicity is very similar for the target rodents and for humans. (Warfarin and other anticoagulant rodenticides were initially developed to overcome this problem by creating compounds that were highly toxic to rodents, particularly after repeated exposures, but much less toxic to humans.) Second, since rodents usually share environments with humans and other mammals, the risk of accidental exposure is an integral part of the placement of baits for the rodents. Finally, as rodents have developed resistance to existing rodenticides, there is a continuous need to develop new and potentially more toxic rodenticides. As rodents have become resistant to warfarin baits, for example, the development of "superwarfarins" has increased the risk to humans.[1,2] It is important to be familiar with use patterns and development of more toxic compounds and to make every effort to identify the actual agent used in order to institute the most appropriate management for these poisonings.

COUMARINS AND INDANDIONES

Toxicology

Warfarin and related compounds (coumarins and indandiones) are the most commonly ingested rodenticides in the United States, with 13,345 exposures reported in 1996.[3] Gastrointestinal absorption of these toxicants is efficient. Warfarin can be absorbed across the skin, but this has occurred only under extraordinary circumstances.

Coumarins and indandiones depress the hepatic synthesis of vitamin K dependent blood–clotting factors (II (prothrombin), VII, IX, and X). The anti-prothrombin effect is best known, and is the basis for detection and assessment of clinical poisoning. The agents also increase permeability of capillaries throughout the body, predisposing the animal to widespread internal hemorrhage. This generally occurs in the rodent after several days of warfarin ingestion due to the long half–lives of the vitamin K dependent clotting factors,[1,2] although lethal hemorrhage may follow smaller doses of the modern, more toxic compounds.[1]

The lengthened prothrombin time (PT) from a toxic dose of coumarins or indandiones may be evident within 24 hours, but usually reaches a maximum in 36–72 hours.[1,4,5] Lengthened PT occurs in response to doses much lower than that necessary to cause hemorrhage. There is concern that the more toxic modern compounds, such as brodifacoum and difenacoum, may cause serious poisoning of nontarget mammals, including humans, at much lower dosage. Brodifacoum, one of the superwarfarins, is much more toxic, with a dose as low as 1 mg in an adult or 0.014 mg/kg in a child sufficient to produce toxicity.[1]

Symptomatic poisoning, with prolonged symptoms due to the long half-lives of superwarfarins, has been reported even with single exposures; however, these are usually intentional and are large single dosages.[2] Because of their toxicity in relation to warfarin, patients may require higher dosages of vitamin K and will require longer monitoring of their PT. One patient required vitamin K for several months following discharge.[6] Another patient was released from the hospital with significant clinical improvement and only slightly elevated coagulation studies after brodifacoum ingestion. Two and a half weeks later, he presented in a comatose state and was found to have massive intracranial hemorrhage.[7]

Clinical effects of these agents usually begin several days after ingestion, due to the long half-life of the factors. Primary manifestations include nosebleeds, bleeding gums, hematuria, melena, and extensive ecchymoses.[1,2,6,7,8] Patients may also have symptoms of anemia, including fatigue and dyspnea on exertion.[8] If the poisoning is severe, the patient may progress to shock and death.

Unlike the coumarin compounds, some indandiones cause symptoms and signs of neurologic and cardiopulmonary injury in laboratory rats leading to death before hemorrhage occurs. These actions may account for the greater toxicity of indandiones in rodents. Neither neurologic nor cardiopulmonary manifestations have been reported in human poisonings.

Confirmation of Poisoning

Coumarin or indandione poisoning results in an increase in prothrombin time, the result of reduced plasma prothrombin concentration. This is a reliable test for absorption of physiologically significant doses. Detectable reduction in prothrombin occurs within 24–48 hours of ingestion and persists for 1–3 weeks.[1,4,5] The manufacturers can often measure blood levels of the more toxic coumarins.[8]

Treatment

1. Determine quantity ingested. If it is certain that the patient ingested no more than a mouthful or two of warfarin- or indandione-treated bait, or a single swallow or less of bait treated with the more toxic brodifacoum or bromadiolone compounds, medical treatment is probably unnecessary.

2. Vitamin K₁. A patient presenting within 24 hours after ingestion will likely have a normal PT. However, in a study of 110 children who were poisoned by superwarfarins, primarily brodifacoum, a child's PT was significantly more likely to be prolonged at 48 hours after having a normal PT at 24 hours.[5] Therefore, for suicidal ingestions with large amounts taken, if there is uncertainty about the amount of bait ingested or the general health of the patient, phytonadione (vitamin K₁) given orally protects against the anticoagulant effect of these rodenticides, with essentially no risk to the patient. In accidental ingestions with healthy children involving only a taste or single swallow, no medical treatment is required, but children should be observed for bleeding and bruising. If a larger amount may have been ingested, PT should be monitored at 24 and 48 hours, with phytonadione therapy initiated for elevated PT or clinical signs of bleeding.

Caution: Phytonadione, specifically, is required. Neither vitamin K₃ (menadione, Hykinone[R]) nor vitamin K₄ (menadiol) is an antidote for these anticoagulants.

Dosage of Phytonadione (oral):

- *Adults and children over 12 years:* 15–25 mg.

- *Children under 12 years:* 5–10 mg.

Alternatively, a colloidal preparation of phytonadione, Aquamephyton[R], may be given intramuscularly. For adults and children over 12 years, give 5–10 mg; for children under 12, give 1–5 mg.

Ensure that patients (especially children) are carefully observed for at least 4–5 days after ingestion. The indandiones and some of the more recently introduced coumarins may have other toxic effects.

---

3. Gastrointestinal decontamination. If large amounts of anticoagulant have been ingested within several hours prior to treatment, consider gastric decontamination procedures as outlined Chapter 2.

4. Determine prothrombin time. If anticoagulant has been ingested any time in the preceding 15 days, determination of the PT provides a basis for judging the severity of poisoning. Patients who ingest large amounts, particularly of the superwarfarin compounds, will likely have a very prolonged period of decreased prothrombin activity. Patients may need to be treated for as long as 3 or 4 months.[6,7]

If the prothrombin time is significantly lengthened, give Aquamephyton[R] intramuscularly. See next page for dosage.

> **Dosage of Aquamephyton^R (intramuscular):**
>
> - *Adults and children over 12 years:* 5-10 mg.
>
> - *Children under 12 years:* 1-5 mg.
>
> Decide dose within these ranges according to the degree of prothrombin time lengthening and, in children, the age and weight of the child. Substantially higher doses of phytonadione (50 to 125 mg) have been required in some poisonings with brodifacoum when bleeding and PT elevation persisted despite therapy.[6,7,9]
>
> Repeat prothrombin time in 24 hours. If it has not decreased from the original value, repeat Aquamephyton^R dosage.

5. Bleeding. If victim is bleeding as a result of anticoagulant poisoning, administer Aquamephyton^R intravenously: up to 10 mg in adults and children over 12 years, and up to 5 mg in children under 12 years. Initial dosage should be decided chiefly on the basis of the severity of bleeding. Subsequent dosages may need to be adjusted based on response, especially in the case of the superwarfarins.[6,7,9] Repeat intravenous Aquamephyton^R in 24 hours if bleeding continues. Inject at rates not exceeding 5% of the total dose per minute. Intravenous infusion of the Aquamephyton^R diluted in saline or glucose solution is recommended. Bleeding is usually controlled in 3-6 hours.

Caution: Adverse reactions, some fatal, have occurred from intravenous phytonadione injections, even when recommended dosage limits and injection rates were observed. For this reason, the intravenous route should be used *only* in cases of severe poisoning. Flushing, dizziness, hypotension, dyspnea, and cyanosis have characterized adverse reactions.

Antidotal therapy in cases of severe bleeding should be supplemented with transfusion of fresh blood or plasma. Use of fresh blood or plasma represents the most rapidly effective method of stopping hemorrhage due to these anticoagulants, but the effect may not endure. Therefore, the transfusions should be given along with phytonadione therapy.

Determine PT and hemoglobin concentrations every 6-12 hours to assess effectiveness of antihemorrhagic measures. When normal blood coagulation is restored, it may be advisable to drain large hematomata.

Ferrous sulfate therapy may be appropriate in the recuperative period to rebuild lost erythrocyte mass.

INORGANIC RODENTICIDES

Toxicology

Thallium sulfate is well absorbed from the gut and across the skin. It exhibits a very large volume of distribution (tissue uptake) and is distributed chiefly to the kidney and liver, both of which participate in thallium excretion. Most blood-borne thallium is in the red cells. Elimination half-life from blood in the adult human is about 1.9 days. Most authors report the LD_{50} in humans to be between 10 and 15 mg/kg.[10]

Unlike other inorganic rodenticides like yellow phosphorus and zinc phosphide, thallium poisoning tends to have a more insidious onset with a wide variety of toxic manifestations. Alopecia is a fairly consistent feature of thallium poisoning that is often helpful diagnostically; however, it occurs two weeks or more after poisoning and is not helpful early in the presentation.[10,11] In addition to hair loss, the gastrointestinal system, central nervous system, cardiovascular system, renal system, and skin are prominently affected by toxic intakes.

Early symptoms include abdominal pain, nausea, vomiting, bloody diarrhea, stomatitis, and salivation. Ileus may appear later on. Elevated liver enzymes may occur, indicating tissue damage. Other patients experience signs of central nervous system toxicity including headache, lethargy, muscle weakness, paresthesias, tremor, ptosis, and ataxia. These usually occur several days to more than a week after exposure.[10,12] Extremely painful paraesthesias, either in the presence or absence of gastrointestinal signs, may be the primary presenting complaint.[11,13] Myoclonic movements, convulsions, delirium, and coma reflect more severe neurologic involvement. Fever is a bad prognostic indication of brain damage.

Cardiovascular effects include early hypotension, due at least in part to a toxic myocardiopathy. Ventricular arrythmias may occur. Hypertension occurs later and is probably a result of vasoconstriction. The urine may show protein and red cells. Patients may also develop alveolar edema and hyaline membrane formation in the lungs, consistent with a diagnosis of Acute Respiratory Distress Syndrome.[14] Death from thallium poisoning may be caused by respiratory paralysis or cardiovascular collapse. Absorption of nonlethal doses of thallium has caused protracted painful neuropathies and paresis, optic nerve atrophy, persistent ataxia, dementia, seizures, and coma.[11]

Yellow phosphorus (also known as white phosphorus) is a corrosive agent and damages all tissues it comes in contact with, including skin and the gut lining. Initial symptoms usually reflect mucosal injury and occur a few minutes to 24 hours following ingestion. The first symptoms include severe vomiting and burning pain in the throat, chest, and abdomen. The emesis may be bloody (either red, brown, or black)[15] and on occasion may have a garlic smell.[16,17] In some cases, central nervous system signs such as lethargy, restlessness, and irritability are the earliest symptoms, followed by symptoms of gastrointestinal injury. Shock and cardiopulmonary arrest leading to death may occur early in severe ingestions.[17]

If the patient survives, a relatively symptom-free period of a few hours or days may occur, although this is not always the case.[15] The third stage of toxicity then ensues with systemic signs indicating severe injury to the liver, myocardium, and brain. This is due to phosphine gas (PH_3) formed in and absorbed from the gut. Nausea and vomiting recur. Hemorrhage occurs at various sites reflecting a depression of clotting factor synthesis in the damaged liver. Also, thrombocytopenia may contribute. Hepatomegaly and jaundice appear. Hypovolemic shock and toxic myocarditis may develop. Brain injury is manifested by convulsions, delirium, and coma. Anuric renal failure commonly develops due to shock and to the toxic effects of phosphorus products and accumulating bilirubin on renal tubules. The mortality rate of phosphorus poisonings may be as high as 50 percent.[15]

Zinc phosphide is much less corrosive to skin and mucous membranes than yellow phosphorus, but inhalation of dust may induce pulmonary edema. The emetic effect of zinc released in the gut may provide a measure of protection; however, phosphine will be produced in the gut and absorbed along with the zinc. Nausea and vomiting, excitement, chills, chest tightness, dyspnea, and cough may progress to pulmonary edema. Patients face many of the same systemic toxicities as encountered with yellow phosphorus, including hepatic failure with jaundice and hemorrhage, delirium, convulsions, and coma (from toxic encephalopathy), tetany from hypocalcemia, and anuria from renal tubular damage. Ventricular arrythmias from cardiomyopathy and shock also occur and are another common cause of death.[16,18] Inhalation of phosphine gas from improper use of phosphide rodenticides has resulted in pulmonary edema, myocardial injury, and multisystem involvement.[19] For more information about the effects of phosphine gas poisoning, see the section on phosphine in Chapter 16, Fumigants.

Confirmation of Poisoning

Phosphorus and phosphides sometimes impart a foul rotten fish odor to vomitus, feces, and sometimes the breath. Luminescence of vomitus or feces is an occasional feature of phosphorus ingestion. Hyperphosphatemia and hypocalcemia occur in some cases, but are not consistent findings.

Thallium can be measured in the serum, urine, and hair. Hair analysis is likely to be useful only in establishing protracted prior absorption. Serum concentration does not exceed 30 mcg per liter in non-exposed persons. The most reliable method for diagnosis is considered a 24-hour urine excretion. The normal value is less than 10 mcg/liter per 24 hours.[10,13]

Treatment: Thallium Sulfate

1. Gastrointestinal decontamination. If thallium sulfate was swallowed less than an hour prior to treatment, consider gastrointestinal decontamination as outlined in Chapter 2. Multiple doses of activated charcoal may be helpful in increasing thallium elimination.[13]

2. Electrolyte and glucose solutions should be given by intravenous infusion to support urinary excretion of thallium by diuresis. Monitor fluid balance carefully to insure that fluid overload does not occur. If shock develops, give whole blood, plasma, or plasma expanders. Pressor amines must be used very carefully in light of myocardial injury. Monitor ECG for arrhythmias.

3. Convulsions. Control seizures and myoclonic jerking as outlined in Chapter 2.

4. Combined hemodialysis and hemoperfusion has proven moderately effective in reducing the body burden of thallium in victims of severe poisoning. In one case, peritoneal dialysis was not effective.

5. Chelation therapy. Several methods for chelating and/or accelerating disposition of thallium have been tested and found either relatively ineffective or hazardous. Chelating agents are not recommended in thallium poisoning. Potassium chloride has been recommended. However it has been reported to increase toxicity to the brain,[11,14] and has not shown to increase elimination in some cases.[20]

6. Potassium ferric ferrocyanide (Prussian Blue) orally enhances fecal excretion of thallium by exchange of potassium for thallium in the gut. It is not available or approved for use in humans in the United States. Reports of its use in humans are anecdotal and do not strongly support its use.

Treatment: Yellow Phosphorus and Zinc Phosphide

1. Skin decontamination. Brush or scrape non–adherent phosphorus from the skin. Wash skin burns with copious amounts of water. Make sure all particles of phosphorus have been removed. If burned area is infected, cover with an antimicrobial creme. See Chapter 2.

2. Supportive management. Poisonings by ingested yellow phosphorus or zinc phosphide are extremely difficult to manage. Treatment is basically supportive and symptomatic. Control of airway and convulsions must be established prior to considering gastrointestinal decontamination as described in Chapter 2.

Caution: Highly toxic phosphine gas may evolve from emesis, lavage fluid, and feces of victims of these poisons. The patient's room should be well ventilated. Persons attending the patient must wear gloves to avoid contact with the phosphorus.

3. Lavage with 1:5000 potassium permanganate solution has been used in the management of ingested phosphorus compounds in the past; however, there is not sufficient evidence for its efficacy and we do not recommend it.

4. Catharsis is probably not indicated, but there may be some benefit in administering mineral oil. Dosage is 100 mL for adults and children over 12 years, and 1.5 mL/kg body weight in children under 12 years. Do not give vegetable oils or fats.

5. Transfusions. Combat shock and acidosis with transfusions of whole blood and appropriate intravenous fluids. Monitor fluid balance and central venous pressure to avoid fluid overload. Monitor blood electrolytes, glucose, and pH to guide choice of intravenous solutions. Administer 100% oxygen by mask or nasal tube.

6. Oxygen. Combat pulmonary edema with intermittent or continuous positive pressure oxygen.

7. Renal protection. Monitor urine albumin, glucose, and sediment to detect early renal injury. Extracorporeal hemodialysis will be required if acute renal failure occurs, but it does not enhance excretion of phosphorus. Monitor ECG to detect myocardial impairment.

8. Liver damage. Monitor serum alkaline phosphatase, LDH, ALT, AST, prothrombin time, and bilirubin to evaluate liver damage. Administer Aquamephyton^R (vitamin K_1) if prothrombin level declines.

9. Pain management. Morphine sulphate may be necessary to control pain. Adult dose: 2-15 mg IM/IV/SC Q 2-6 hours prn. Child's dose: 0.1-0.2 mg/kg/dose Q 2-4 hours.

10. Phosphine gas. For specific therapy due to phosphine gas, refer to the treatment of phosphine poisoning in Chapter 16, Fumigants.

CONVULSANTS

Toxicology

Crimidine is a synthetic chlorinated pyrimidine compound that, in adequate dosage, causes violent convulsions similar to those produced by strychnine.

Sodium fluoroacetate and fluoroacetamide are readily absorbed by the gut, but only to a limited extent across skin. The toxic mechanism is distinct from that of fluoride salts. Three molecules of fluoroacetate or fluoroacetamide are combined in the liver to form a molecule of fluorocitrate, which poisons critical enzymes of the tricarboxylic acid (Krebs) cycle, blocking cellular respiration. The heart, brain, and kidneys are the organs most prominently affected. The effect on the heart is to cause arrhythmias, progressing to ventricular fibrillation, which is a common cause of death. Metabolic acidosis, shock, electrolyte imbalance, and respiratory distress are all poor prognostic signs. Neurotoxicity is expressed as violent tonic-clonic convulsions, spasms, and rigor, sometimes not occurring for hours after ingestion.[21]

Strychnine is a natural toxin (nux vomica) which causes violent convulsions by direct excitatory action on the cells of the central nervous system, chiefly the spinal cord. Death is caused by convulsive interference with pulmonary function, by depression of respiratory center activity, or both. Strychnine is detoxified in the liver. Residence half-life is about 10 hours in humans. Onset of symptoms is usually within 15-20 minutes of ingestion. Lethal dose in adults is reported to be between 50 and 100 mg, although as little as 15 mg can kill a child.[22]

Confirmation of Poisoning

There are no generally available tests to confirm poisoning by the convulsant rodenticides.

Treatment: Sodium Fluoroacetate and Fluoroacetamide

Poisonings by these compounds have occurred almost entirely as a result of accidental and suicidal ingestions. If the poison was ingested shortly before treatment and convulsions have not yet occurred, the first step in treatment is to remove the toxicant from the gut. If the victim is already convulsing, however, it is necessary first to control the seizures before gastric lavage and catharsis are undertaken.

1. Control seizures as outlined in Chapter 2. Seizure activity from these compounds may be so severe that doses necessary for seizure control may paralyze respiration. For this reason, it is best to intubate the trachea as early as

CONVULSANTS

crimidine
  Castrix
fluoroacetamide*
  Compound 1081
sodium fluoroacetate
  Compound 1080
strychnine

* Discontinued in the U.S.

Only specially trained personnel are allowed to use strychnine. Crimidine and sodium fluoroacetate are no longer registered for use as pesticides.

possible in the course of seizure control, and support pulmonary ventilation mechanically. This has the added advantage of protecting the airway from aspiration of regurgitated gastric contents.

2. Gastrointestinal decontamination. If the patient is seen within an hour of exposure and is not convulsing, consider gastrointestinal decontamination as outlined in Chapter 2.

3. Administer intravenous fluids cautiously to support excretion of absorbed toxicant. It is especially important to avoid fluid overload in the presence of a weak and irritable myocardium.

4. Monitor electocardiogram for arrhythmias and, if detected, treat with an appropriate antiarrhythmic drug. Facilities for electroshock cardioversion should be at hand. Some victims of fluoroacetate poisoning have been rescued after repeated cardioversions.

5. Calcium gluconate (10% solution) given slowly intravenously should be given to relieve hypocalcemia. Care must be taken to avoid extravasation.

Dosage of Calcium Gluconate:

Supplied as 100 mg/mL (10% solution)

- *Adults and children over 12 years:* 10 mL of 10% solution, given slowly, intravenously. Repeat as necessary.

- *Children under 12 years:* 200-500 mg/kg/24 hr divided Q6 hr. For cardiac arrest, 100 mg/kg/dose. Repeat dosage as needed.

---

6. Other therapies. Antidotal efficacy of glycerol monacetate and ethanol, observed in animals, has not been substantiated in humans. These therapies are not recommended in humans.

Treatment: Strychnine or Crimidine

Strychnine and crimidine cause violent convulsions shortly following ingestion of toxic doses. Both poisons are probably well adsorbed onto charcoal. If the patient is seen fully conscious and not convulsing a few moments after the ingestion, great benefit may derive from the immediate ingestion of activated charcoal. If the patient is already obtunded or convulsing, the involuntary motor activity must be controlled before steps are taken to empty the gut and limit toxicant absorption.

1. Control seizures as outlined in Chapter 2.

2. Gastrointestinal decontamination. Consider gastrointestinal decontamination if patient is seen within an hour of ingestion.

3. Administer intravenous fluids to support excretion of absorbed toxicants. Inclusion of sodium bicarbonate in the infusion fluid counteracts metabolic acidosis generated by convulsions. Effectiveness of hemodialysis and hemoperfusion has not been tested.

MISCELLANEOUS RODENTICIDES: RED SQUILL AND CHOLECALCIFEROL

Toxicology

Red squill is a little-used rodenticide, consisting of the inner portions of a small cabbage plant grown in eastern Mediterranean countries. Its toxic properties have been known since ancient times and are probably due to cardiac glycosides. For several reasons, mammals other than rodents are unlikely to be poisoned: (1) red squill is intensely nauseant, so that animals which vomit (rodents do not) are unlikely to retain the poison; (2) the glycoside is not efficiently absorbed from the gut; and (3) absorbed glycoside is rapidly excreted. Injection of the glycosides leads to effects typical of digitalis: alterations in cardiac impulse conduction and arrhythmias.

Cholecalciferol is the activated form of vitamin D (vitamin D_3). Its toxic effect is probably a combination of actions on liver, kidney, and possibly the myocardium, the last two toxicities being the result of hypercalcemia. Early symptoms and signs of vitamin D-induced hypercalcemia in humans are fatigue, weakness, headache, and nausea. Polyuria, polydipsia, proteinuria, and azotemia result from acute renal tubular injury by hypercalcemia. This is commonly the cause of death. Prolonged hypercalcemia results ultimately in nephrolithiasis and nephrocalcinosis. Azotemia occurs as renal tubular damage progresses.

Confirmation of Poisoning

Cholecalciferol intoxication is indicated by an elevated concentration of calcium (chiefly the unbound fraction) in the serum. There are no generally available tests for the other rodenticides or their biotransformation products.

Treatment: Red Squill

Red squill is unlikely to cause poisoning unless ingested at substantial dosage. The problem is usually self-correcting due to its intense emetic effect. If, for some reason, the squill is retained, syrup of ipecac, followed by 1-2 glasses of water, should be administered to initiate vomiting. Monitor cardiac status electrocardiographically.

Treatment: Cholecalciferol

Cholecalciferol at high dosage may cause severe poisoning and death. Human poisonings from its use as a rodenticide have not been reported, but vitamin D overdosage has occurred under clinical circumstances. Treatment is directed at limiting gastrointestinal absorption, accelerating excretion, and counteracting the hypercalcemic effect.

1. Gastrointestinal decontamination. If cholecalciferol has been ingested within an hour prior to treatment, consider gastric decontamination, as outlined in Chapter 2. Repeated administration of charcoal at half or more the initial dosage every 2-4 hours may be beneficial.

2. Administer intravenous fluids (normal saline or 5% glucose) at moderate rates to support excretory mechanisms and excretion. Monitor fluid balance to avoid overload, and measure serum electrolytes periodically. Measure total and ionized calcium levels in the blood 24 hours after cholecalciferol ingestion to determine severity of toxic effect. Monitor urine for protein, and red and white cells to assess renal injury.

3. Furosemide (Lasix), 20-40 mg intravenously, or 40-120 mg daily by mouth may be given to promote diuresis. Dosage for children under 12 is approximately 0.5-1.0 mg/kg body weight intravenously, 1.0-2.0 mg/kg body weight orally. Monitor serum potassium after dosage; give potassium chloride if hypokalemia occurs. Consult package insert for additional directions and warnings.

4. Predinisone and similar glucocorticoids reduce elevated blood calcium levels in certain diseases. Although they have not been tested in cholecalciferol overdosage, it is possible that they would be beneficial. Dosage is approximately 1 mg per kilogram per day, to a maximum of 20 mg per day.

5. Calcitonin (salmon calcitonin, Calcimar[R]) is a logical antidote for cholecalciferol actions, but has only very limited use in human poisoning.[23] In other conditions, the usual dosage is 4 International Units per kg body weight every 12 hours, by intramuscular or subcutaneous injection, continued for 2-5 days.

The dose may be doubled if calcium-lowering effect is not sufficient. Calcium gluconate for intravenous injection should be immediately available if indications of hypocalcemia (carpopedal spasm, cardiac arrhythmias) appear. Consult package insert for additional directions and warnings.

6. Cholestryamine appears effective in the treatment of vitamin D toxicity in animals.[24] It has seen very limited use in humans.[25,26]

References

1. Mack RB. Not all rats have four legs: Superwarfarin poisoning. *N C Med J* 1994;55:554-6.

2. Katona B and Wason S. Superwarfarin poisoning. *J Emerg Med* 1989;7:627-31.

3. Litovitz TL, Smilkstein M, Felberg L, et al. 1996 Annual Report of the American Association of Poison Control Centers Toxic Exposure Surveillance System. *Am J Emerg Med* 1997;15:447-500.

4. Burucoa C, Mura P, Robert R, et al. Chlorophacinone intoxication. *Clin Toxicol* 1989;27:79-89.

5. Smolinske SC, Scherger DL, Kearns PS, et al. Superwarfarin poisoning in children: A prospective study. *Pediatrics* 1989;84:490-4.

6. Lipton RA and Klass EM. Human ingestion of a 'superwarfarin' rodenticide resulting in a prolonged anticoagulant effect. *JAMA* 1984;252:3004-5.

7. Helmuth RA, McCloskey DW, Doedens DJ, et al. Fatal ingestion of a brodifacoum-containing rodenticide. *Lab Med* 1989;20:25-7.

8. Norcross WA, Ganiats TG, Ralph LP, et al. Accidental poisoning by warfarin-contaminated herbal tea. *West J Med* 1993;159:80-2.

9. Kruse JA and Carlson RW. Fatal rodenticide poisoning with brodifacoum. *Ann Emerg Med* 1992;21:331-6.

10. Mayfield SR, Morgan DP, and Roberts RJ. Acute thallium poisoning in a 3-year old child. *Clin Pediatr (Phila)* 1983;23:461-2.

11. Bank WJ, Pleasure DE, Suzuki K, et al. Thallium poisoning. *Arch Neurol* 1972;26:456-64.

12. Fred HL and Accad MF. Abdominal pain, leg weakness, and alopecia in a teenage boy. *Hosp Pract* 1997;32:69-70.

13. Meggs WJ, Hoffman RS, Shih RD, et al. Thallium poisoning from maliciously contaminated food. *J Toxicol Clin Toxicol* 1994;32:723-30.

14. Roby DS, Fein AM, Bennett RH, et al. Cardiopulmonary effects of acute thallium poisoning. *Chest* 1984;85:236-40.

15. McMarron MM and Gaddis GP. Acute yellow phosphorus poisoning from pesticide pastes. *Clin Toxicol* 1981;18:693-711.

16. Dipalma JR. Human toxicity from rat poison. *Am Fam Physician* 1981;24:186-9.

17. Simon FA and Pickering LK. Acute yellow phosphorus poisoning: Smoking stool syndrome. *JAMA* 1976;235:1343-4.

18. Patial RK, Bansal SK, Kashyap S, et al. Hypoglycaemia following zinc phosphide poisoning. *J Assoc Physicians India* 1990;38:306-7.

19. Schoonbroodt D, Guffens P, Jousten P, et al. Acute phosphine poisoning? A case report and review. *Acta Clin Belg* 1992;47:280-4.

20. Koshy KM and Lovejoy FH. Thallium ingestion with survival: Ineffectiveness of peritoneal dialysis and potassium chloride diuresis. *Clin Toxicol* 1981;18:521-5.

21. Chi CH, Chen KW, Chan SH, et al. Clinical presentation and prognostic factors in sodium monofluoroacetate intoxication. *Clin Toxicol* 1996;34:707-12.

22. Benomran FA and Henry JD. Homicide by strychnine poisoning. *Med Sci Law* 1996;36:271-3.

23. Buckle RM, Gamlen TR, and Pullen IM. Vitamin D intoxication treated with procine calcitonin. *Br Med J* 1972;3:205-7.

24. Queener SF and Bell NH. Treatment of experimental vitamin D3 intoxication in the rat with cholestyramine. *Clin Res* 1976;24:583A.

25. Jibani M and Hodges NH. Prolonged hypercalcaemia after industrial exposure to vitamin D. *Br Med J* 1985;290:748-9.

26. Thomson RB and Johnson JK. Another family with acute vitamin D intoxication: Another cause of familial hypercalcaemia. *Postgrad Med J* 1986;62:1025-8.

CHAPTER 18

Miscellaneous Pesticides, Solvents, and Adjuvants

There are a variety of pesticides that do not fall into the broad categories described in other chapters in this manual. Many of them are widely used and are therefore associated with a high probability of human exposure. Some have significant toxicity as well as a likelihood of human exposure, and are of real concern. Many of the solvents and adjuvants used in the formulation of pesticides also present a high likelihood of human exposure. Such exposures can result in significant toxic effects that in many cases exceed the toxicity of the active pesticide ingredient(s). Furthermore, it is sometimes more difficult to obtain information about the solvents and adjuvants, complicating the issues of diagnosis and management.

4-AMINOPYRIDINE

Toxicology

4-Aminopyridine is a highly toxic white powder used as a bird repellent. It works by making one or two birds acutely ill, thus warning off the remaining birds by cries of distress. It is toxic to all vertebrates.[1] It is usually added to grain baits in 0.5%–3.0% concentration, but 25% and 50% concentrates in powdered sugar are available. Recent human exposure has come from its use as an investigational drug in the treatment of multiple sclerosis.[2,3] It is rapidly absorbed by the gut, less effectively across skin. The chief mechanism of toxicity is enhancement of cholinergic transmission in the nervous system through the release of acetylcholine both centrally and peripherally. Due to enhanced transmission at neuromuscular junctions, severe muscle spasms may be a prominent manifestation of toxicity.[2] 4-Aminopyridine is rapidly metabolized and excreted.

No human poisonings have occurred as a result of ordinary use, but the effects of ingestion of about 60 mg each by two adults have been reported. Both experienced immediate abdominal discomfort, nausea and vomiting, weakness, dizziness, and profuse diaphoresis, and one went on to develop a tonic–clonic seizure and required ventilatory support. Acidosis was present in both cases.[1] Dizziness, giddiness, and gait disturbances are common, and seizures may be severe, although recovery with supportive therapy and ventilatory support has been the usual outcome.[1,2,3]

HIGHLIGHTS

- Physicians may need to actively seek information from producers regarding exact makeup of "inert ingredients"

Signs and Symptoms:

- Highly variable based on agent
- Many are irritants and corrosives
- Creosote (phenolic compounds) give a smoky color to urine
- Methemoglobinemia may occur with sodium chlorate and creosote poisoning
- Sodium chlorate also causes renal injury, arrhythmia, shock, and DIC
- Pneumonitis occurs with hydrocarbon aspiration

Treatment:

- Skin, eye, and GI decontamination
- Supportive care and seizure control
- Methylene blue for methemoglobinemia

Treatment

1. Skin decontamination. If skin or eye contamination has occurred, thorough washing of the skin or eyes is indicated. See Chapter 2.

2. Gastrointestinal decontamination. If the patient is seen within an hour of ingestion of a significant quantity of this compound, gastrointestinal decontamination should be considered, as outlined in Chapter 2. If treatment is delayed, immediate oral administration of charcoal and sorbitol may represent reasonable management.

3. Seizures may require anticonvulsant medication. See Chapter 2 for dosages.

4. Muscular spasms. Neuromuscular blockade with drugs such as d–tubocuarine, metocurine and pancuronium bromide have been used sucessfully to relieve the muscular spasms that occur with this agent. Such therapy must be provided in an intensive care setting.[1]

5. Dehydration should be treated with intravenous fluids if oral fluids cannot be retained.

CALCIUM CYANAMIDE

This synthetic compound is marketed as granules containing 44% calcium cyanamide, yielding 19.5% nitrogen. It is incorporated into soil to serve as fertilizer, fungicide, and herbicide. In contact with water, hydrogen cyanamide is released. Acidic conditions accelerate this reaction. Hydrogen cyanamide is a solid with considerable vapor pressure. It has toxic properties totally different from those of cyanide, and it does not degrade to cyanide.

Toxicology

Calcium cyanamide is only moderately irritating to skin, but hydrogen cyanamide is severely irritating and caustic to skin and the inhaled gas is strongly irritating to mucous membranes.[4] Dermal and mucosal lesions in the mouth, tongue, and upper esophagus have occurred after exposure. No systemic symptoms from dermal exposure have been reported.[5] Systemic poisonings have followed inhalation of hydrogen cyanamide and ingestion of the salt. Manifestations of poisoning include flushing, headache, vertigo, dyspnea, tachycardia, and hypotension, sometimes progressing to shock.[4] Because cyanamide is an inhibitor of acetaldehyde dehydrogenase, ingestion of alcohol exaggerates the symptoms. (A citrated form of cyanamide has been used in place of Antabuse in alcohol aversion therapy.)

Treatment

1. Skin decontamination. Skin contamination with either the calcium salt or the free form should be removed by washing with soap and water. Flush eyes with copious amounts of clean water. If skin or eye irritation persists, medical attention should be obtained promptly. See Chapter 2.

2. Gastrointestinal decontamination. If large doses have been ingested within an hour of exposure, gastrointestinal decontamination should be considered. If dosage was small or treatment is delayed, oral administration of activated charcoal and sorbitol probably represents reasonable management. See Chapter 2 for doses.

3. Hypotension or Antabuse-type reactions should be treated by placing the patient in the Trendelenburg position, giving intravenous fluids, including plasma or blood, if needed, and, if necessary, vasopressor drugs parenterally.

4. Atropine is not antidotal.

CREOSOTE

Creosote is obtained by distillation of the tar formed by heating wood or coal in the absence of oxygen. It is purified by extraction into oils. Creosote from wood consists mainly of guaiacol (methoxy phenol) and cresol (methyl phenol). Coal-derived creosote contains, in addition, some phenol, pyridine, and pyridinol. Creosote is extensively used as a wood preservative, usually by high-pressure impregnation of lumber. It has also been used as an animal dip and disinfectant. Much of human exposure is in the form of various phenol compounds.

Creosote is irritating to skin, eyes, and mucous membranes. Workers in contact with technical creosote or with treated timbers sometimes develop skin irritation, vesicular or papular eruptions, dermal pigmentation, and occasionally gangrene and skin cancer.[6] Photosensitization has been reported. Eye contamination has resulted in conjunctivitis and keratitis, sometimes resulting in corneal scarring. The constituents of creosote are efficiently absorbed across the skin, but systemic poisonings following dermal absorption have occurred very rarely. Absorption of ingested creosote from the gut occurs promptly, and there may be significant absorption of vapor by the lung. Conjugates of absorbed phenolic constituents are excreted mainly in the urine. Acute toxic effects are similar to those of lysol, but the corrosive nature of creosote is somewhat less because of greater dilution of phenol in the creosote.[7] Irritation of the gastrointestinal tract, toxic encephalopathy, and renal tubular injury are the principal effects. A chronic toxicosis from continuing gastrointestinal absorption (creosote used medicinally) has been described, consisting of gastroenteritis and visual disturbances.

Manifestations of acute systemic poisoning are salivation, vomiting, dyspnea, headache, dizziness, loss of pupillary reflexes, cyanosis, hypothermia, convulsions, and coma. Death is due to multi-organ system failure as patients develop shock, acidosis, respiratory depression, and anuric renal failure.

Confirmation of Poisoning

The presence of phenolic oxidation products imparts a dark, smoky color to the urine.[7] If there is suspicion of poisoning, addition of a few drops of ferric chloride solution to the urine yields a violet or blue color, indicating the presence of phenolic compounds.

Treatment

1. Skin decontamination. Stringent measures should be taken to avoid contamination of skin or eyes and inhalation of vapor. Skin contamination should be promptly washed off with soap and water. Remove eye contamination by washing with copious amounts of water, then obtain specialized medical attention promptly because corneal injury may be severe. See Chapter 2.

2. Gastrointestinal decontamination. If a significant amount of creosote has been ingested and the patient is alert and able to swallow, immediately administer a slurry of activated charcoal by mouth. Further efforts to limit absorption will depend on whether there has been corrosive injury to the esophagus. If pharyngeal redness and swelling are evident, neither induced emesis nor gastric lavage is advisable due to potential re-exposure of the esophagus to the creosote, or perforation of the esophagus from a gastric tube. For further information on gastric decontamination, including charcoal dosing, see Chapter 2.

3. Maintain pulmonary ventilation mechanically with oxygen, if necessary.

4. Blood and urine samples. Draw a blood sample to test for methemoglobinemia, to measure BUN and blood electrolytes, and to check for signs of liver injury (bilirubin, GGT, LDH, ALT, AST, and alkaline phosphatase). Examine the urine for protein and cells, and for "smoky" phenolic excretion products.

5. Intravenous fluids. Give fluids intravenously to correct dehydration and electrolyte disturbances. Include glucose to protect the liver and bicarbonate to relieve metabolic acidosis, as necessary. Monitor fluid balance carefully to signal discontinuation of intravenous fluids if renal failure occurs. Plasma or blood transfusion may be needed to overcome shock.

6. Monitor ECG to detect arrhythmias and/or conduction defects that may appear as manifestations of a toxic myocardiopathy.

7. Convulsions. Anticonvulsants may be needed to control seizures as outlined in Chapter 2.

8. Hemodialysis is not effective in accelerating disposition of phenol (or, presumably, creosote), but hemoperfusion over charcoal probably is effective.[8] This should be considered in severe creosote poisonings.

9. Methemoglobinemia is rarely severe, but intravenous administration of 1% methylene blue may be considered if 25-30% of hemoglobin is converted. Dose is 0.1 mL of 1% solution per kg body weight, given over no less than 10 minutes. Nausea, dizziness, and a transient increase in blood pressure may occur.

ENDOTHALL

As the free acid or as sodium, potassium, or amine salts, endothall is used as a contact herbicide, defoliant, aquatic herbicide, and algacide. It is formulated in aqueous solutions and granules at various strengths.

Toxicology

Endothall is irritating to the skin, eyes, and mucous membranes. It is well absorbed across abraded skin and from the gastrointestinal tract. Recognized systemic toxic mechanisms in mammals are: corrosive effects on the gastrointestinal tract (particularly from high concentrations of the free acid); cardiomyopathy and vascular injury leading to shock; and central nervous system injury, causing convulsions and respiratory depression. A single case has been reported of lethal poisoning in a previously healthy 21-year-old man who died after ingestion of 7-8 grams of endothall. In this patient, hemorrhage and edema were noted in the gastrointestinal tract and lungs.[9] There are no standards for levels, and they are not considered useful in management.

Treatment

1. Skin decontamination. Wash endothall from the skin with soap and water. Flush contamination from the eyes with copious amounts of clean water. Obtain medical attention if irritation of skin or eyes persists. See Chapter 2.

2. Gastrointestinal decontamination. If a large quantity has been ingested, the patient is seen within an hour of exposure, and is fully alert and not convulsing, gastrointestinal decontamination should be considered as outlined in Chapter 2. Lavage is usually contraindicated due to the corrosive nature of this agent.

3. Intubation. If there are indications of corrosive effects in the pharynx, gastric intubation should not be attempted because of the risk of esophageal perforation. Treatment procedures appropriate for ingestions of corrosives (strong acids and alkalis) may be necessary. Referral should be made to a surgeon or gastroenterologist for consideration of endoscopy.

4. Oxygen should be given by mask. If respiratory drive is weak, pulmonary ventilation may have to be supported mechanically.

5. Monitor blood pressure closely. Infusions of plasma, blood, other volume expanders, and pressors may be needed to combat shock.

6. Administer intravenous fluids to correct dehydration, stabilize electrolytes, provide sugar, and support mechanisms for toxicant disposition. Give vasoactive amines very carefully in light of possible myocardiopathy.

7. Convulsions. Seizures may require administration of diazepam and/or other anticonvulsants.

8. Hemodialysis. It is not known whether hemodialysis or hemoperfusion would be effective in removing endothall from the blood. This option should be considered if the patient's condition deteriorates despite supportive care.

METALDEHYDE

Toxicology

Metaldehyde is a four-unit cyclic polymer of acetaldehyde which has long been used to kill slugs and snails, which are attracted to it without the use of bait. Occasional poisonings of animals and children have resulted from ingestion of pellets intended as molluscicide, but tablets designed as a combustible fuel ("meta-fuel") have also been responsible for human poisonings.[10] Another form of exposure is "snow storm tablets," which the user places at the end of a lighted cigarette to create snow. Toxicity occurs through inhalation of metaldehyde fumes.[11] The biochemical mechanism of poisoning is not known. Both acetaldehyde and metaldehyde produced similar effects in dogs; however, acetaldehyde was not detected in the plasma or urine of the metaldehyde-poisoned dogs.[12]

Ingestion of a toxic dose is often followed shortly by nausea and vomiting. The other primary features of toxicity are pyrexia, generalized seizures, and mental status changes, sometimes leading to coma.[10,13] Other signs and symptoms that may occur include hypersalivation, facial flushing, dizziness, tachypnea, and acidosis.[10,11] Pneumonitis has followed inhalational exposure to metaldehyde.[11] While most cases are dramatic with significant seizures and coma, fatal events are infrequent.[10,13] Poisoned animals show tremors, ataxia, hyperesthesia, salivation, ataxia, and seizures.[12] Autopsy findings in fatal human poisonings indicate severe damage to liver cells and renal tubular epithelium.

Confirmation of Poisoning

Metaldehyde can be measured in the blood and urine, although there are very few reports of levels among poisoned humans. One patient who had severe tonic clonic seizures and was comatose had a metaldehyde level in the serum of 125 mg/L with a half-life of 27 hours. This patient did not have detectable acetaldehyde in the serum.[13]

Treatment

1. Gastrointestinal decontamination. If ingestion occurred within an hour of treatment, consider gastrointestinal decontamination as outlined in Chapter 2. Activated charcoal may well be useful against metaldehyde.

2. Convulsions. If seizures occur, sedative anticonvulsants must be administered. See Chapter 2 for dosage.

3. Supportive treatment. Appropriate supportive treatment including intravenous fluids containing saline and glucose should be given. Sodium bicarbonate may be considered in the event of severe metabolic acidosis. Fluid balance and electrolytes must be monitored carefully to avoid fluid overload if renal failure supervenes.

4. Renal failure. There is no specific antidote for metaldehyde poisoning. Hemodialysis is probably not effective in removing metaldehyde, but must be instituted if renal failure occurs. The effectiveness of hemoperfusion has not been tested.

5. Liver function tests and urine sediment examination should be done to assess liver and kidney injury in poisoned patients.

SODIUM CHLORATE

Sodium chlorate is used in agriculture as a defoliant, nonselective contact herbicide, and semipermanent soil sterilant. Because of its explosive nature, it must be formulated with water-soluble fire retardant material, such as sodium metaborate, soda ash, magnesium chloride, or urea. It is usually applied in water solution.

Toxicology

Sodium chlorate is irritating to skin, eyes, and mucous membranes of the upper respiratory tract.[14] Dermal absorption is slight. Even though gastrointestinal absorption is also inefficient, severe (sometimes fatal) poisoning follows ingestion of a toxic dose, estimated at about 20 grams in the adult human. Excretion is chiefly in the urine. The principal mechanisms of toxicity are hemolysis, methemoglobin formation, cardiac arrhythmia (partly secondary to hyperkalemia), and renal tubular injury.[14,15]

The irritant action on the gut causes nausea, vomiting, and abdominal pain. Once absorbed, hemoglobin is rapidly oxidized to methemoglobin, and intravascular hemolysis occurs.[14] Cyanosis is prominent if methemoglobinemia is severe and may be the only presenting sign.[15] Acute tubular necrosis and hemoglobinuria may result from the hemolysis or direct toxic injury. Plasma and urine are dark brown from the presence of free hemoglobin and methemoglobin.[14,15,16] Release of potassium from red cell destruction results in hyperkalemia which may be severe enough to cause life-threatening arrythmias.[16] The liver and spleen are often enlarged due to uptake of hemolyzed erythrocytes.[15] Hypoxemia may lead to convulsions. Death may be the result of shock, tissue hypoxia, renal failure, hyperkalemia, or disseminated intravascular coagulation (DIC).[14,15,16]

Confirmation of Poisoning

There are no widely available tests specifically for chlorate. Dark brown staining of the plasma and urine indicates the action of a strong oxidizing agent on hemoglobin. See Chapter 2.

Treatment

1. Skin decontamination. Skin contamination should be removed immediately by washing with soap and water. Medical attention should be sought if irritation persists. Flush contamination from eyes with copious amounts of clean water, then obtain specialized medical attention promptly, because irritant action may be severe. See Chapter 2.

2. Gastrointestinal decontamination. If sodium chlorate has been ingested within an hour prior to treatment, consider gastrointestinal decontamination as outlined in Chapter 2.

3. Oxygen. If respiration is depressed, ventilatory support may be necessary.

4. Sodium thiosulfate has been recommended as an antidote against absorbed sodium chlorate. Thiosulfate is thought to inactivate the chlorate ion to form the less toxic chloride ion. It can be given orally or as an IV infusion over 60-90 minutes. The dose is 2-5 g dissolved in 200 mL of 5% sodium bicarbonate.[14]

5. Monitor blood pressure, fluid balance, blood electrolytes, BUN, methemoglobin, and bilirubin, as well as urine protein, cells and free hemoglobin content, and ECG. Widening of the QRS complex and prolongation of the PR interval indicate hyperkalemic cardiac toxicity.

6. Milk may be helpful in relieving the pain of gastric irritation.

7. Administer intravenous fluids to sustain chlorate excretion. Maintain urine pH in the alkaline range by adding sodium bicarbonate to the infusion fluid. Monitor urine production closely, so that intravenous fluids can be slowed or discontinued if renal failure occurs. Blood transfusion may be needed if hemolysis and methemoglobinemia are severe. Exchange transfusion has been recommended to enhance clearance and treat DIC.[16]

8. Hemodialysis may be life-saving in severe poisoning. It is effective in removing chlorate from the blood, provides a means to control hyperkalemia, and makes possible the control of extracellular fluid volume and composition while renal function remains impaired.

9. Methemoglobinemia. Administration of methylene blue to reverse methemoglobinemia may be considered if as much as 25-30% of hemoglobin is converted. Give intravenously 0.1 mL/kg body weight of a 1% solution over a period of at least 10 minutes. An increase in blood pressure, nausea, and dizziness may occur, but these effects are usually transient. As the use of this agent in chlorate poisoning has not proven beneficial in the past, it is still advisable to proceed to exchange transfusion as stated in #7.

SYNERGISTS: PIPERONYL BUTOXIDE

Synergists are chemical agents included in pesticide products to enhance the killing power of the active ingredients. The widely-used insecticide synergist, piperonyl butoxide, acts by inhibiting the enzymatic degradation of pyrethrins, rotenone, N-methyl carbamates, and possibly some other insecticides. There is limited dermal absorption on contact. Inherent toxicity in mammals is low. Large absorbed doses may theoretically enhance the toxic hazard of the rapidly metabolized insecticides used today, although inhibition of human drug-metabolizing enzymes by these agents has not actually been demonstrated. Their presence in pesticide products to which humans are exposed does not change the basic approach to management of poisoning, except that some possibility of enhanced toxicity of the active insecticidal ingredients should be kept in mind.

SOLVENTS AND ADJUVANTS

Liquid materials in which pesticides are dissolved and the solids on which they are adsorbed (sometimes called carriers or vehicles) are selected by producers to achieve stability of the active ingredient, convenience in handling and application, and maximum killing power following application. Often, the particular solvents and adjuvants selected by pesticide manufacturers are responsible for giving their commercial products a competitive edge. For this reason, their inclusion in marketed products is usually proprietary information, not available to the general public except in emergencies. If a poisoning emergency exists, pesticide companies will usually cooperate in supplying physicians with information needed to provide treatment. Some companies will put the inert ingredients on the Material Safety Data Sheet (MSDS). The physician should seek this information to assist in evaluating all possible exposures. A direct request to the producer is the quickest way to secure this information. Physicians may also contact EPA directly for this information (tel: 703-305-7090) if needed for proper management of a case.

Petroleum distillates are the most commonly used solvents for lipophilic pesticides. Most insecticides are lipophilic. The distillates are mixtures of aliphatic and aromatic hydrocarbons and have low boiling points.

Sometimes specific **hydrocarbons,** such as toluene or xylene (strongly odiferous), are added to stabilize the solution of insecticide or make it more emulsifiable. Hydrocarbon-dissolved pesticides are usually diluted for application by adding measured amounts of water to form emulsions. Some chlorinated hydrocarbons may be present in particular technical mixtures. A strong odor lingering after application of a structural pest control spray is often due to the solvent rather than the active ingredient.

Less lipophilic active ingredients are sometimes dissolved in mixtures of alcohols, glycols, ethers, or various chlorinated solvents. It is possible that these enhance the dermal absorbability of some pesticides. Some solvents, such as methanol and isopropanol, may represent a significant toxic hazard if swallowed in sufficient dosage.

Granular formulations utilize various clay materials which adsorb pesticide, retain it in more or less stable form until application, then desorb the material slowly into treated soil. There is some significant desorption when granules are in contact with human skin and very substantial desorption into gastrointestinal secretions if granules are swallowed. The clay materials themselves are not a toxic hazard.

Dusts are infrequently used today. Various forms of talc (silicatecarbonate particles) have been used in the past to adsorb pesticides for application to foliage. Particle sizes are such that these dusts are usually trapped in the upper respiratory mucous when inhaled. When the mucous is swallowed, the particles desorb pesticide into gastrointestinal secretions. Dust formulations may, therefore, release enough of some pesticides to cause systemic poisonings.

Stickers and spreaders (film extenders) are organic substances added to formulations to disperse pesticide over treated foliage surfaces and enhance adhesion. The availability and persistence of residue on the leaf surfaces is thereby increased. Substances used include proteinaceous materials (milk products, wheat flour, blood albumin, gelatin), oils, gums, resins, clays, polyoxyethylene glycols, terpenes, and other viscid organics. Some also include sulfated alcohols, fatty acid esters, and alkyl and petroleum sulfonates. For persons exposed in the course of formulation or application of pesticides, these adjuvants probably add little or no toxic hazard to that inherent in the active pesticidal ingredients.

Emulsifiers serve to stabilize water-oil emulsions formed when water is added to technical hydrocarbon concentrates. Chemically, they resemble detergents (one part of the molecule lipophilic, the other hydrophilic). Long-chain alkyl sulfonate ethers of polyethylene glycol and polyoxyethylene oleate are exemplary emulsifiers. They have low inherent mammalian toxicity, and their presence probably has little effect on the overall toxicity of formulated products which include them.

Penetrants facilitate the transfer of herbicide from foliage surface to the interior tissues. Some are lipids while others are detergent (surfactant) in nature. Substances used include heavy petroleum oils and distillates, polyol fatty acid esters, polyethoxylated fatty acid esters, aryl alkyl polyoxyethylene glycols, alkyl amine acetate, alkyl aryl sulfonates, polyhydric alcohols, and alkyl phosphates. Some of these are eye and skin irritants, and may account for the irritant effects of particular herbicide formulations whose active ingredients do not have this property.

Safeners are substances added to mixtures of fertilizers with pesticides (commonly herbicides) to limit the formation of undesirable reaction products. Some substances used are alcohol sulfates, sodium alkyl butane diamate, polyesters of sodium thiobutane dioate, and benzene acetonitrile derivatives. Some are moderately irritating to the skin and eyes. Systemic toxicities are generally low.

Anticaking agents are added to granular and dust formulations to facilitate application by preventing cakes and clumps. Among several products used are the sodium salt of mono- and di-methyl naphthalene sulfonate, and diatomaceous earth. Diatomaceous earth has little adverse effect except a drying action on the skin. Methyl naphthalenes are said to be skin irritants and photosensitizers; whether their derivatives have this effect is not known.

Treatment

Petroleum distillates are mineral hydrocarbons which undergo limited absorption across the gut. In general, clinical toxicologists do not recommend induced emesis or gastric lavage in treating ingestions of these materials, because of the serious risk of hydrocarbon pneumonitis if even tiny amounts of the liquid are aspirated into the lung. However, this injunction against emptying the stomach may be set aside when the petroleum distillate is a vehicle for toxic pesticides in significant concentration. In such cases, if the patient is seen within one hour of exposure, gastrointestinal decontamination should be considered.

Rapid respiration, cyanosis, tachycardia, and low-grade fever are the usual indications of frank hydrocarbon pneumonitis. Patients with presumed hydrocarbon pneumonitis, who are symptomatic, should usually be hospitalized, preferably in an intensive care setting. If the patient has pulmonary symptoms, a chest x-ray should be taken to detect or confirm signs of pneumonitis. In addition, the urine should be examined for protein, sugar, acetone, casts, and cells, and an ECG should be examined for arrhythmias and conduction defects. Mechanically assisted pulmonary ventilation with 100% oxygen may be required. Hydrocarbon pneumonitis is sometimes fatal, and survivors may require several weeks for full recovery. In milder cases, clinical improvement usually occurs within several days, although radiographic findings will remain abnormal for longer periods.[17]

The presence of chlorinated solvents in some formulations may add significantly to the toxic hazard, particularly if the product is ingested. Certain adjuvants are irritants to skin, eyes, and mucous membranes, and may account for the irritant properties of some products whose active ingredients do not have this effect. With these exceptions, however, the presence of adjuvants in most finished pesticide products probably does not enhance or reduce systemic mammalian toxicity to any great extent.

References

1. Spyker DA, Lynch C, Shabanowitz J, et al. Poisoning with 4-aminopyridine: Report of three cases. *Clin Toxicol* 1980;16:487-97.

2. Pickett TA and Enns R. Atypical presentation of 4-aminopyridine overdose. *Ann Emerg Med* 1996;27:382-5.

3. Stork CM and Hoffman RS. Characterization of 4-aminopyridine in overdose. *Clin Toxicol* 1994;32:583-7.

4. Sittig M. Handbook of Toxic and Hazardous Chemicals and Carcinogens, 3rd ed. Park Ridge, NJ: Noyes Publications, 1991, pp. 316-7.

5. Torrelo A, Soria C, Rocamora A, et al. Lichen planus-like eruption with esophageal involvement as a result of cyanamide. *J Am Acad Dermatol* 1990;23:1168-9.

6. Sittig M. Handbook of Toxic and Hazardous Chemicals and Carcinogens, 3rd ed. Park Ridge, NJ: Noyes Publications, 1991, pp. 450-3.

7. Bowman CE, Muhleman MF, and Walters E. A fatal case of creosote poisoning. *Postgrad Med J* 1984;60:499-500.

8. Christiansen RG and Klaman JS. Successful treatment of phenol poisoning with charcoal hemoperfusion. *Vet Hum Toxicol* 1996;38:27-8.

9. Allender WJ. Suicidal poisoning by endothall. *J Anal Toxicol* 1983;7:79-82.

10. Longstreth WT and Pierson DJ. Metaldehyde poisoning from slug bait ingestion. *West J Med* 1982;137:134-7.

11. Jay MS, Kearns GL, Stone V, et al. Toxic pneumonitis in an adolescent following exposure to snow storm tablets. *J Adolesc Health* 1988;9:431-3.

12. Booze TF and Oehme FW. An investigation of metaldehyde and acetaldehyde toxicities in dogs. *Fundam Appl Toxicol* 1986;6:440-6.

13. Moody JP and Inglis FG. Persistence of metaldehyde during acute molluscicide poisoning. *Hum Exp Toxicol* 1992;11:361-2.

14. Helliwell M and Nunn J. Mortality in sodium chlorate poisoning. *Br Med J* 1979;1:1119.

15. Steffen C and Seitz R. Severe chlorate poisoning: Report of a case. *Arch Toxicol* 1981;48:281-8.

16. Smith EA and Oehme FW. A review of selected herbicides and their toxicities. *Vet Hum Toxicol* 1991;33:596-608.

17. Anas N, Namasonthi V, and Ginsburg CM. Criteria for hospitalizing children who have ingested products containing hydrocarbons. *JAMA* 1981;246:840-3.

Disinfectants

HIGHLIGHTS

- Compounds are registered for medical or medicinal use rather than as pesticides
- Several are among the most frequently reported human poisonings in the U.S.
- Iodine is well absorbed through abraded or burned skin

Signs and Symptoms:

- Highly variable based on agent
- Many are irritants and corrosives
- Iodine causes neurological symptoms, shock, renal failure, and hyperkalemia
- Pine oil can cause aspiration pneumonia

Treatment:

- Follow general principles of decontamination and supportive care

Contraindicated:

- Gastric emptying and decontamination procedures are contraindicated in poisonings due to corrosive agents and pine oil

A wide variety of disinfectant agents are used to destroy microorganisms and they differ greatly in their toxic effects. Most disinfectants can conveniently be grouped into a few categories, some of which are also represented in other classes of pesticides. Many of these materials are not registered as pesticides, but are registered for medical or medicinal use. This chapter reviews a few of the more common or more severely toxic disinfectants.

ALCOHOLS

Alcohols have a long history of use as disinfectants. Often disinfectants are mixtures, usually of ethanol and isopropyl alcohol (isopropanol). The alcohol most commonly used in households as a disinfectant is isopropyl alcohol, commonly marketed as a 70% solution. It is a clear, colorless liquid with an odor similar to ethanol.

Toxicology of Isopropyl Alcohol

Isopropyl alcohol is well and rapidly absorbed from the gastrointestinal tract. It is also well absorbed by skin and by inhalation. It is considered to be more toxic to the central nervous system than ethanol, with similar effects. Both ingestion and inhalation at high concentrations can result in the rapid onset of CNS depression with subsequent coma and death. Apnea commonly accompanies this CNS depression.[1,2] Similar neurological toxicity has been reported with excessive topical exposure to the umbilicus of a neonate.[3] Irritation of the gastrointestinal tract results in gastritis and severe vomiting. Isopropyl alcohol may also produce mild hepatic injury with acute exposures. Acute tubular necrosis has been reported with this agent,[1] but the renal toxicity is not as great as with methanol poisonings. Ketosis without metabolic acidosis but prominent hypoglycemia is common.[2,3] This ketosis is the result of direct metabolism of this compound to acetone.[1,3] Monitoring of isopropyl levels is useful, when available. In addition, blood levels of acetone and glucose should be determined to aid in management.

Confirmation of Poisoning

Isopropyl alcohol can be measured in the blood and urine. Serum acetone can also be measured. Blood isopropyl alcohol levels of 128-200 mg/dL have been associated with death.

Treatment: Isopropyl Alcohol

1. Gastrointestinal decontamination. Since the onset of coma is often rapid with this poisoning, induced emesis is contraindicated, though spontaneous vomiting often occurs. If the patient has ingested a large amount, has not vomited, and is seen within one hour of exposure, consideration should be given to gastric emptying by lavage as outlined in Chapter 2.

Isopropyl alcohol is well adsorbed to charcoal, so activated charcoal should probably be administered, as outlined in Chapter 2.

2. Supportive care for hypotension and respiratory depression is critical to survival and should be administered whenever possible in an intensive care setting.

3. If **hypoglycemia** occurs, glucose administration is indicated in order to maintain normoglycemia.

4. Hemodialysis has been reported to be beneficial in patients with severe poisoning unresponsive to standard supportive therapy.[1,4]

ALDEHYDES

The two aldehydes most commonly used as disinfectants are formaldehyde and glutaraldehyde. Formaldehyde is discussed in Chapter 17, Fumigants. Glutaraldehyde is very similar to formaldehyde in its toxicity and treatment, although it is probably slightly less toxic. Glutaraldehyde is commonly prepared as an aqueous solution at a 2% concentration, and is slightly alkaline in this solution. It has been reported to cause respiratory irritation, resulting in rhinitis[5,6] and occupational asthma.[6,7,8] It has also resulted rarely in palpitations and tachycardia in human subjects. At high dosage, given orally, it results in gastrointestinal irritation with diarrhea, which may be hemorrhagic. Due to the irritant effects of glutaraldehyde, the wearing of personal protective equipment is required for the protection of skin (29 CFR 1910.132), and eyes (29 CFR 1910.133). OSHA standards require the use of appropriate respirators by employees that may be exposed to glutaraldehyde during routine or emergency work procedures (29 CFR 1910.134).

Commercial Products

ALCOHOLS
isopropyl alcohol

ALDEHYDES
formaldehyde
glutaraldehyde

CATIONIC DETERGENTS
benzalkonium chloride
cetrimide
cetylpyridium chloride

CHLORHEXIDINE
Hibiclens
Hibistat
Peridex

HYPOCHLORITES
calcium hypochlorite
sodium hypochlorite

IODINES
povidone-iodine
Betadine
Ioprep
Pharmadine

MERCURIALS
mercurobutol
mercurochrome
merthiolate
nitromersol
phenylmercuric acetate
phenylmercuric nitrate
thimerosol

PHENOLS
2-benzyl-4-chlorophenol
cresol
Lysol
hexachlorophene
Bilevon
Dermaadex
Exofene
Gamophen
Phisohex
Surgi-Cen
Surofene
Texosan
o-phenylphenol
phenol
4-tert-amylphenol
thymol
triclosan

PINE OIL

Treatment: Glutaraldehyde

1. Gastrointestinal decontamination. If a large amount has been ingested and retained, and the patient is seen within one hour of exposure, consider gastric emptying as described in Chapter 2. Administration of activated charcoal should be considered, as described in Chapter 2.

2. Oxygen. If patient has been in an area with strong odor of glutaraldehyde due to vaporization, remove to fresh air area and administer oxygen as needed.

3. Skin decontamination. If skin irritation is noted, vigorous skin decontamination is indicated. However, systemic toxicity from skin exposure appears unlikely.

CATIONIC DETERGENTS

Several cationic detergents are used as disinfectants. All share the capacity, in sufficient concentration, to behave as caustic agents, capable of causing rather severe, caustic burns. It appears that concentrations greater than approximately 7.5% are necessary to produce significant caustic injuries. However, experience with human exposures to these compounds is very limited. The three agents most commonly used as detergent disinfectants are benzalkonium chloride, cetrimide, and cetylpyridium chloride.

Though there are no cetrimide preparations available in the U.S., several are available in European Union countries. Concentrated solutions are usually only available in industrial settings, such as production of consumer products, or for use in hospitals for disinfectant purposes. Therefore, acute poisonings are uncommon.

Toxicology

In low-concentration solutions, these agents have been reported to cause eye discomfort as well as skin rashes and irritation. In stronger concentrations, they can cause severe corneal and skin burns. Likewise, strong concentrations will result in caustic burns to lips, oral mucosa, esophagus, and stomach.[9,10] Vomiting, diarrhea, and abdominal pain have been reported.[11] Necrosis of the gut, with peritonitis, has also been reported.[12] In severe exposures, there are also reports of CNS depression, liver injury, and pulmonary edema.[9,11]

Treatment

1. Skin decontamination. If a high-concentration solution has been applied to skin, aggressive skin contamination and treatment of burns is appropriate. If a high concentration solution is in contact with the eyes, profuse washing of the eyes is indicated followed by a careful exam of the corneas. If burns have occurred, appropriate ophthalmologic care should be provided.

2. Gastrointestinal decontamination. Gastric emptying and other methods of gastrointestinal decontamination are **contraindicated** in these poisonings. Some experts recommend cautious dilution with small amounts of milk or water.[9,13] Acidic solutions such as juices should never be offered for dilution.

3. Endoscopy. If a highly concentrated solution was ingested or oral burns are noted, the patient needs urgent endoscopy for grading of the caustic injury. The endoscopy should be performed within 24 hours to minimize the risk of perforation from the procedure.[12] A competent surgeon or gastroenterologist should provide subsequent care.

4. Other agents. Although corticosteroids are commonly used to treat these burns, their use remains controversial. Use of other agents, such as H2 antagonists and sulcralfate, has been reported but remains controversial at this time.

5. CNS, pulmonary and other systemic effects should be treated symptomatically, consistent with sound medical practice.

CHLORHEXIDINE

Chlorhexidine is a cationic biguanide, available in concentrations up to 4% as a topical agent used as a skin cleanser and mouthwash. Skin preparations of 0.5%-4% are marketed under the trade names Hibiclens[R] and Hibistat[R]. It is also marketed as a mouthwash in a 0.12% solution under the trade name Peridex[R]. There is very little human experience with poisonings, as these concentrations do not appear to be significantly toxic.

Toxicology

Chlorhexidine is poorly absorbed from skin or the gastrointestinal tract. Therefore most effects noted have been primarily local. If a low concentration solution is ingested or applied to the skin, mild local irritation can be seen. Contact dermatitis, urticaria, and anaphylaxis have followed repeated skin exposures to this agent.[14,15] Corneal injuries have been described in several cases after inadvertent exposure of the eyes to the 4% concentration. These injuries have resulted in permanent corneal scarring.[16] Esophageal burns have been reported in a single case after ingestion of a large quantity of a 20% solution of this agent.[17] Ulcerative colitis has been described after an enema of the 4%

solution mixed with tap water (10 mL in 2 liters water).[18] Liver toxicity can occur with large exposures.[17]

Treatment

1. Gastrointestinal decontamination. If ingestion of a large quantity has occurred within an hour and the patient has not vomited, gastrointestinal decontamination as described in Chapter 2 should be considered. If a highly concentrated solution has been ingested, manage as a caustic ingestion as described in the cationic detergents, without gastrointestinal decontamination.

2. Liver injury panel should be performed with large ingestions.

3. Eye decontamination. If eye exposure has occurred, the eyes should be vigorously irrigated and a careful ophthalmologic exam should be performed for corneal injury. If an injury has occurred, an ophthalmologic consultation should be obtained.

HYPOCHLORITES

Hypochlorites are implicated in a large proportion of the disinfectant poisonings reported to poison control centers in the United States. Most are solutions of sodium or calcium hypochlorite solutions. Chloramine, a disinfectant used by many municipal water supplies, is an infrequent cause of acute poisonings. Sodium and calcium hypochlorite solutions are of relatively low toxicity. They are mildly corrosive to the eyes,[19] and mucous membrane burns have been reported.[20] Significant poisonings are very infrequent with these agents in solution.[21]

When hypochlorite solutions are mixed with acids or ammonia solutions, chlorine or chloramine gas is produced, resulting in an irritant with pulmonary toxicity. Many brief exposures have led to transient symptoms requiring limited emergency department management.[22] However, in cases of prolonged exposure or exposure to high concentrations, there is the potential for severe toxic pneumonitis.[23] While severe injury may be the exception to the rule, great efforts should be made to discourage mixing of these materials with acid or ammonia.

Treatment

1. Gastric decontamination. After oral exposures, gastric emptying is not indicated. If a granular material is ingested, and the patient has symptomatic mucosal burns, referral to a surgeon or gastroenterologist for consideration of endoscopy and management may be appropriate.

2. **Dilution** with water or milk not to exceed approximately 15 mL/kg in a child or 120-240 mL in an adult is probably appropriate if vomiting has not occurred. Administration of acids is contraindicated, due to the risk or increasing generation of chlorine gas.

3. **Eye decontamination.** If eyes were exposed, they should be irrigated profusely with water or saline. If corneal burns are detected, referral to an ophthalmologist is appropriate.

4. **Skin decontamination.** Skin exposure should also be managed by copious water dilutions. See Chapter 2.

5. **Fresh air.** If exposure to vapors or chlorine or chloramine gas has occurred, patient should immediately be moved to fresh air. If symptoms occur or persist, oxygenation should be assessed and oxygen should be administered as needed. If persistent symptoms occur, a chest film should be obtained and hospital care considered. Intensive care may need to be provided in severe inhalations.

IODINE

The most common iodine-containing disinfectant is povidone-iodine (proviodine), in 7.5-10% solutions. Povidone-iodine is described as an iodophor, which is a complex of iodine and polyvinylpyrrolidone, a solubilizing agent. It is intended to liberate free iodine in solution for its effect. Although reported concentrations of iodine in these solutions is only 80-120 ugm/dL, the total available iodine is approximately 10% of the povidone-iodine. Therefore a 10% solution will have in the range of 1% total available iodine.

Toxicology of Povidone-Iodine

This compound is very poorly absorbed from the gastrointestinal tract, due to the rapid conversion of free iodine to iodide in the stomach. Although highly concentrated iodine solutions or iodine salts are corrosive to the gastrointestinal tract,[24] solutions of povidone-iodine have little caustic potential. Likewise, the compound is poorly absorbed from intact skin. All symptomatic poisonings reported have occurred either after repeated exposure to burned skin, or following irrigation of wounds, joints, or serosal surfaces such as the mediastinum.[25-28] The one exception was an infant who received an enema of povidone-iodine in a polyethylene glycol solution, followed by whole bowel irrigation with polyethylene glycol mixed with povidone-iodine. This child died with severe hyperglycemia and very high iodine levels.[24]

In povidone-iodine exposures by these routes, the primary symptoms initially appear to be neurological, with headache, dizziness, delirium, hallucinations, and seizures.[26] Hypotension, arrythmias, cyanosis, metabolic acidosis, shock, and acute renal failure occur in severe cases.[25,27,28] Hepatic injury, manifested by elevated serum transaminase levels, has also been reported with very high level exposures.[27] Hyperkalemia has occurred, and the serum chloride may be falsely elevated due to the presence of a second halide.[25]

Treatment: Povidone-Iodine

1. Skin decontamination. Remove skin contamination by vigorous washing with soap and water. See Chapter 2.

2. Gastrointestinal decontamination. If the patient is seen soon after a very large ingestion, and vomiting has not occurred, consider gastrointestinal decontamination, as outlined in Chapter 2. Consider single dose charcoal.

3. Iodine clearance is apparently enhanced by procedures that enhance chloride excretion. Therefore, osmotic or choluretic diuresis is probably indicated in these poisonings, if symptomatic.

4. Seizures. Treat seizures with anticonvulsants, as outlined in Chapter 2.

5. Monitor thyroid function following recovery to confirm euthyroid state.

MERCURIALS

A wide variety of organic mercurials have been used as disinfectants and as preservatives. Nearly all uses have been banned in the United States. The toxicity and treatment of exposure to these compounds is described in detail in Chapter 15, Fungicides, under organomercury compounds and will not be repeated here.

PHENOLS

Several phenols are used as disinfectants. Cresol and thymol are alkyl derivatives of phenol, while hexachlorophene and triclosan are chlorinated phenols. Common commercial preparations are Lysol[R], a 50% solution of mixed cresols in soap, and hexachlorophene, marketed under several trade names in soap bars and some cosmetics. Cresols and hexachlorophene are discussed individually as examples of these compounds that are familiar and for which there are some human data.

Toxicology of Cresols

Cresols, in common with phenol and other phenolic compounds, are highly corrosive to all surfaces. With ingestion of concentrated forms they cause severe corrosive injury to the mouth and upper gastrointestinal tract. Likewise, severe eye and skin caustic injuries can occur with cresol exposure.[29] Symptoms usually include nausea, vomiting, and diarrhea. Hypotension, myocardial failure, pulmonary edema, and neurological changes may also occur.[30] Liver and renal toxicity, methemoglobinemia, and hemolysis have all been reported.[30,31] After long-term, repeated exposure, contact dermatitis may complicate these exposures. These compounds are well absorbed from the gastrointestinal tract and are also significantly absorbed from the skin and by inhalation.

Treatment: Cresols

1. Gastrointestinal decontamination. Due to the corrosive nature of these compounds, gastrointestinal decontamination should not be attempted. Consideration of dilution with milk or water is appropriate if vomiting has not occurred.

2. Endoscopy. If a corrosive injury has occurred with burns to the mouth, or if there is a clear history of gastrointestinal exposure, endoscopy should be considered and a gastroenterologist or surgeon should be consulted for diagnosis and management.

3. Skin decontamination. If skin or eye contamination has occurred, copious irrigation should be performed. This should be followed by a careful eye examination for corneal burns. If corneal burns are noted, ophthalmologic consultation should be obtained.

4. Respiratory and circulatory support should be provided in accordance with sound medical management. If severe systemic symptoms persist, the patient should be treated in an intensive care unit, if possible.

Toxicology of Hexachlorophene

Hexachlorophene is well absorbed orally and dermally. Dermal exposures have led to severe toxicity and death in neonates, due to application to damaged skin, or repeated or high-concentration skin exposures.[32] Hexachlorophene should never be used as a disinfectant on open wounds or abraded or inflamed skin surfaces. In distinction to other phenolic compounds, this agent is not significantly caustic and exposure does not result in the severe caustic injuries seen with other phenolic chemicals.

Hexachlorophene is a potent neurotoxicant. It causes brain edema and spongy degeneration of white matter.[33] This neurotoxicity can be seen after acute or chronic exposures, either by skin absorption or ingestion. The nervous system symptoms are complex. Lethargy is an early manifestation, followed by muscular weakness, muscular fasciculation, irritability, cerebral edema, and paralysis, leading to coma and death. Seizures commonly occur in more severe cases.[32,34] Blindness and optic atrophy have been reported following exposure to hexachlorophene.[35]

In addition to the neurological effects, common early symptoms of poisoning are vomiting, diarrhea, and anorexia.[34] These findings have been accompanied in animals by significant hepatotoxicity.[36] With skin exposure, an erythematous desquamative rash is often noted at the site of exposure.[34] With chronic exposure, contact dermatitis may be noted. In severe poisonings, cardiovascular symptoms, including hypotension and bradycardia, have been noted.[37] In a single case, repeated exposure to this compound led to asthma in a pediatric nurse.[38]

Treatment: Hexachlorophene

1. Gastrointestinal decontamination. Since this agent is not generally caustic, consideration should be given to aggressive gastrointestinal decontamination. If the patient has ingested a significant amount and is seen within one hour of exposure, gastric emptying is likely to be useful, as described in Chapter 2.

Since hexachlorophene is thought to have an enterohepatic recirculation, it is possible that repeated dosing of activated charcoal, as outlined in Chapter 2, will enhance clearance of this compound. However, hexachlorophene does not bind well to charcoal and there are no clinical trials of this therapy for this agent.

2. Other therapies. Though this compound is quite toxic systemically and enhanced clearance methods would appear beneficial, there is no evidence to support the efficacy of hemodialysis, peritoneal dialysis, hemoperfusion, or exchange transfusion.[37]

3. Skin decontamination. If exposure has occurred through the skin, aggressive washing of skin with soap or detergent and water is probably beneficial, to remove any residues still on the skin. Since hexachlorophene is not soluble in water, water washing alone will provide no significant benefit. See Chapter 2.

4. Neurological support and control of seizures is critical to survival and should be performed, when possible, in an intensive care setting. Seizure control should be in accordance with recommendations in Chapter 2.

5. Cardiovascular and respiratory support are also very important to success in treating severe poisonings with this agent and should be provided in an intensive care unit in accordance with accepted medical practice.

PINE OIL

Pine oil detergent and disinfectant solutions are among the most common poisonings reported to poison control centers in the U.S. A relatively high number of these are reported as serious or fatal. Pine oil is found in a variety of household and commercial cleaners and disinfectants. It is a mixture of mono-terpenes derived from the distillation of wood from various pine species, with approximately 57% being alpha-pinene.[39] Its most common side effects in smaller dosage are irritation of mucous membranes, gastrointestinal irritation, mild respiratory and CNS depression, and renal toxicity. Larger ingestions can result in severe respiratory distress, cardiovascular collapse, and severe CNS effects. Renal failure and myoglobinuria have also been reported in severe poisonings.[40] Since even small ingestions can result in severe aspiration pneumonia, all ingestions should be considered potentially hazardous.

While many of the reported effects of poisoning with this agent are related to direct irritant effect on mucous membranes, gastrointestinal tract, and lung (by aspiration), some reports suggest significant absorption from oral and rectal exposures. Other reports suggest a lesser rate of absorption.[39] While alpha-terpineol can be measured in blood, there are no data relating levels to degree of toxicity. Consequently, this measure is not considered useful in guiding diagnosis and management.

Treatment

1. Gastrointestinal decontamination. Since there is a high risk of aspiration pneumonia, induced emesis is usually considered contraindicated in these poisonings. However, spontaneous emesis may occur due to direct irritation of the gastric mucosa.

If the patient is seen within an hour of ingestion and a large amount has been ingested, gastric emptying by intubation and lavage may be considered, as described in Chapter 2. However, some studies have suggested greater rates of complications with lavage than with ipecac-induced emesis.[40]

There is no evidence that activated charcoal is helpful in these poisonings. Likewise, though a variety of enhanced elimination methods have been proposed and tried, there is no evidence to support their efficacy.

2. Eye decontamination. If eye exposure has occurred, copious irrigation of the eyes is appropriate.

3. Pulmonary symptoms. The patient should be observed for at least six hours with any significant ingestion in order to observe the onset of any symptoms, particularly pulmonary symptoms. If any pulmonary symptoms are observed, the patient should have a chest film and measurement of oxygenation, and hospitalization is appropriate. With severe pulmonary symptoms, transfer to an intensive care unit is usually appropriate. With severe aspiration, management should be handled as in any severe aspiration pneumonia, in accordance with accepted medical practice. Other severe systemic effects should be treated in accordance with accepted medical practice.

References

1. Lacouture PG, Wason S, Abrams A, et al. Acute isopropyl alcohol intoxication: Diagnosis and management. *Am J Med* 1983;75:680-6.

2. Rich J, Scheife RT, Katz N, et al. Isopropyl alcohol intoxication. *Arch Neurol* 1990;47:322-4.

3. Vivier PM, Lewander WJ, Martin HF, et al. Isopropyl alcohol intoxication in a neonate through chronic dermal exposure: A complication of a culturally-based umbilical care practice. *Pediatr Emerg Care* 1994;10:91-3.

4. Manring E, Meggs W, Pape G, et al. Toxicity of an intravenous infusion of isopropyl alcohol. *J Toxicol Clin Toxicol* 1997;35:503.

5. Norback D. Skin and respiratory symptoms from exposure to alkaline glutaraldehyde in medical services. *Scand J Work Environ Health* 1988;14:366-71.

6. Corrado OJ, Osman J, and Davies RJ. Asthma and rhinitis after exposure to glutaraldehyde in endoscopy units. *Hum Toxicol* 1986;5:325-8.

7. Chan-Yeung M, McMurren T, Catonio-Begley F, et al. Occupational asthma in a technologist exposed to glutaraldehyde. *J Allergy Clin Immunol* 1993; 91(5):974-8.

8. Stenton SC, Beach JR, Dennis JH, et al. Glutaraldehyde, asthma, and work – a cautionary tale. *Occup Med* 1994;44(2):95-8.

9. Mucklow ES. Accidental feeding of a dilute antiseptic solution (chlorhexidine 0.05% with cetrimide 1%) to five babies. *Hum Toxicol* 1988;7:567-9.

10. Wilson JT and Burr IM. Benzaldonium chloride poisoning in infant twins. *AJDC* 1975;129:1208-9.

11. Chan TY. Poisoning due to savlon (cetrimide) liquid. *Hum Exp Toxicol* 1994;13:681-2.

12. Zargar SA, Kochhar R, Mehta S, et al. The role of fiberoptic endoscopy in the management of corrosive ingestion and modified endoscopic classification of burns. *Gastrointest Endosc* 1991;37:165-9.

13. Consensus: POISINDEX[R] Editorial Board consensus opinion poll, Irritants/Caustics Specialty Board. Englewood, CO: Micromedex, 1988.

14. Wong WK, Goh CL, and Chan KW. Contact urticaria from chlorhexidine. *Contact Dermatitis* 1990;22:52.

15. Okano M, Nomura M, Hata S, et al. Anaphylactic symptoms due to chlorhexidine gluconate. *Arch Dermatol* 1989;125:50-2.

16. Tabor E, Bostwick DC, and Evans CC. Corneal damage due to eye contact with chlorhexidine gluconate. *JAMA* 1989;261:557-8.

17. Massano G, Ciocatto E, Rosabianca C, et al. Striking aminotransferase rise after chlorhexidine self-poisoning. *Lancet* 1982;1:289.

18. Hardin RD and Tedesco FJ. Colitis after hibiclens enema. *J Clin Gastroenterol* 1986;8:572-5.

19. Ingram TA. Response of the human eye to accidental exposure to sodium hypochlorite. *J Endod* 1990;16:235-8.

20. French RJ, Tabb HJ, and Rutledge LJ. Esophogeal stenosis produced by ingestion of bleach. *South Med J* 1970;63:1140-4.

21. Landau GD and Saunders WH. The effect of chlorine bleach on the esophagus. *Arch Otolaryngol* 1964;80:174-6.

22. Mrvos R, Dean BS, Krenzelok EP, et al. Home exposure to chlorine/chloramine gas: review of 216 cases. *South Med J* 1993;86:654-7.

23. Reisz GR and Gammon RS. Toxic penumonitis from mixing household cleaners. *Chest* 1986:89:49-52.

24. Kurt TL, Hnilica V, Bost R, et al. Fatal iatrogenic iodine toxicity in a 9-week old infant. *Vet Hum Toxicol* 1992;34:333.

25. Means LJ, Rescorla FJ, and Grosfield JL. Iodine toxicity: An unusual cause of cardiovascular collapse during anesthesia in an infant with Hirschsprung's Disease. *J Pediatr Surg* 1990;25:1278-9.

26. Ponn RB. Continuous povidone-iodine irrigation (letter). *Ann Thorac Surg* 1987;43:239.

27. Pietsch J and Meakins JL. Complications of povidne-iodine absorption in topically treated burn patients. *Lancet* 1976;7:280-2.

28. Campistol JM, Cipiano A, Nogué S, and Bertrán A. Acute renal failure in a patient treated by continuous povidone-iodine mediastinum irrigation. *J Pediatr Surg* 1988;29:410-2.

29. Pegg SP and Campbell DC. Children's burning due to cresol. *Burns* 1985;11:294-6.

30. Arthus GJ, Wise CC, and Coles GA. Poisoning by cresol. *Anaesthesia* 1977;32:642-3.

31. Chan TK, Mak LW, and Ng RP. Methemoglobinemia, heme bodies, and acute massive intravascular hemolysis in lysol poisoning. *Blood* 1971;38:739-44.

32. Mullick FG. Hexachlorophene toxicity – Human experience at the Armed Forces Institute of Pathology. *Pediatrics* 1973;51(2)II:395-9.

33. Anderson JM, Cockburn F, Forfar J, et al. Neonatal spongioform myelinopathy after restricted application of hexachlorophane skin disinfectant. *J Clin Pathol* 1981;34:25-9.

34. Martin-Bouyer G, Lebreton R, Toga M, et al. Outbreak of accidental hexachlorophene poisoning in France. *Lancet* 1982;1:91-5.

35. Slamovitz TL, Burde RM, and Klingele TG. Bilateral optic atrophy caused by chronic oral ingestion and topical application of hexachlorophene. *Am J Ophthalmol* 1980;89:676-9.

36. Prasad GV, Rajendra W, and Indira K. Brain ammonia metabolism in hexachlorophene-induced encephalopathy. *Bull Environ Contam Toxicol* 1987;38:561-4.

37. Boehm RM and Czajka PA. Hexachlorophene poisoning and the ineffectiveness of peritoneal dialysis. *J Toxicol Clin Toxicol* 1979;14(3);257-62.

38. Nagy L and Orosz M. Occupational asthma due to hexachlorophene. *Thorax* 1984;39:630-1.

39. Koppel C, Tenczer J, Tennesmann U, et al. Acute poisoning with pine oil - Metabolism of monoterpenes. *Arch Toxicol* 1981;49:73-8.

40. Litovitz TL, Schmidz BF, Matyunas N, et al. 1987 Annual Report of the American Association of Poison Control Centers National Data Collection System. *Am J Emerg Med* 1988;6:479-515.

Section V

INDEXES

Index of Signs and Symptoms

Presented in this chapter are lists of pesticides reported to have caused particular symptoms and signs, or combinations thereof, in poisoned individuals. The lists may help direct the attention of health professionals to possible toxic causes of the various disease manifestations, prompting inquiry into likelihood of exposure to the listed chemicals. If certain agents appear suspect, inquiry can then be made into the presence of additional manifestations typical of poisoning by those substances.

The limitations of this approach to diagnosis must be understood. First, all manifestations of illness have multiple causes, pesticidal and nonpesticidal. Second, there are no specific symptoms or signs that are invariably present in poisonings by particular pesticides. Third, many poisonings are characterized by unexpected manifestations.

Finally, neither route of exposure nor dosage of pesticide is taken into account in this listing. For example, effects of high-dose ingestion are not distinguished from effects of relatively low-dose dermal absorption, nor are topical effects distinguished from systemic dermal manifestations. The lists of pesticides can only be regarded as *clues* to prompt further inquiry by the interviewing professional.

The term manifestation means either symptom or sign. The word "poisoning" is used loosely in these headings to include topical as well as systemic effects. Pesticides which are relatively consistent in causing particular manifestations are listed in the middle column, headed "Characteristic of These Agents." Pesticides that have caused various conditions with less consistency, or are less prominent features of poisoning, are listed in the right-hand column, headed "Occurs with These Agents." Obviously, the distinction is not clear-cut.

Some symptoms (malaise, fatigue, dizziness) occur so commonly in poisoned individuals that they have little or no value in differential diagnosis, and are therefore not included in these tables.

General

MANIFESTATION	CHARACTERISTIC OF THESE AGENTS	OCCURS WITH THESE AGENTS
Rotten egg odor	Sulfur	
Hypothermia	Creosote Norbormide	
Hyperthermia (fever, pyrexia)	Nitrophenols Pentachlorophenol	Borate Thallium Metaldehyde Inorganic arsenicals Chlorophenoxy compounds Cadmium dusts Naphthalene
Chills	Phosphine Arsine	
Hot sensations	Nitrophenols Chlordimeform	Pentachlorophenol
Myalgia	Paraquat Chlorophenoxy compounds	
Thirst	Pentachlorophenol Nitrophenois Inorganic arsenicals Phosphorus Phosphides Sodium fluoride Cholecalciferol Aminopyridine	Borate Endothall
Anorexia	Organophosphates Carbamate insecticides Nicotine Pentachlorophenol Hexachlorobenzene Chlordimeform Cholecalciferol	Halocarbon fumigants Nitrophenols Inorganic arsenicals Aminopyridine
Alcohol intolerance	Thiram Calcium cyanamide	
Sweet taste in the mouth	Chlordimeform	
Metallic taste in the mouth	Inorganic arsenicals Organic mercury	
Salty, soapy taste In the mouth	Sodium fluoride	

Skin

MANIFESTATION	CHARACTERISTIC OF THESE POISONINGS	OCCURS WITH THESE AGENTS
Irritation, Rash, Blistering, or Erosion (without sensitization)	Copper, organotin, cadmium compounds Metam sodium Paraquat Diquat Sodium chlorate Phosphorus Sulfur Glyphosate Propargite Sodium hypochlorite Quaternary ammonia Thiram Chlordimeform Cationic detergents Hexachlorphene Ethylene oxide Formaldehyde Acrolein Methyl bromide Ethylene dibromide Dibromochloropropane Dichloropropane Endothall Aliphatic acids	Pentachlorophenol Picloram Chlorophenoxy compounds Captan Rotenone Diethyltoluamide Creosote Fungicides Herbicides with irritant properties Petroleum distillate
Contact dermatitis	PCP Paraquat DEET Chlorhexidine Creosote Hexachlorphine Pyrethrins Chlorothalonil Thiram Thiophthalimides	
Flushing	Cyanamide Nitrophenols	Thiram plus alcohol
Dermal sensitization	Propachlor Propargite Ethylene oxide	Anflazine Chlorothalonil Barban Captafol Formaldehyde
Beefy red palms, soles	Borate	
Urticaria	Chlorhexidine PCP DEET	Fluoride Pentachlorophenol
Bullae	Liquid fumigants	Hexachlorobenzene

Skin (continued)

MANIFESTATION	CHARACTERISTIC OF THESE POISONINGS	OCCURS WITH THESE AGENTS
Pallor	Organochlorines Fumigants Sodium fluoride Creosote	Coumarins Indandiones

Cyanosis	Sodium chlorate
	Paraquat
	Cadmium dusts
	Sodium fluoroacetate
	Strychnine
	Crimidine
	Nicotine
	Organochlorines
		Organophosphates
		Carbamate insecticides
		Agents that cause shock,
		  myocardiopathy, severe
		  arrhythmias or convulsions

Yellow stain	Nitrophenols	
Keratoses, brown discoloration	Inorganic arsenicals	
Ecchymoses	Coumarins Indandiones	Phosphorus Phosphides
Jaundice	Carbon tetrachloride Chloroform Phosphorus Phosphides Phosphine Paraquat Sodium chlorate	Inorganic arsenicals Diquat Copper compounds
Excessive hair growth		Hexachlorobenzene
Loss of hair	Thallium	Inorganic arsenicals
Loss of fingernails		Paraquat Inorganic arsenicals
Brittle nails, white striations		Inorganic arsenicals Thallium
Sweating, diaphoresis	Organophosphates Carbamate insecticides Nicotine Pentachlorophenol Naphthalene Aminopyridine	Copper compounds

Eye

MANIFESTATION	CHARACTERISTIC OF THESE POISONINGS	OCCURS WITH THESE AGENTS
Conjunctivitis (irritation of mucous membranes, tearing)	Copper compounds Organotin compounds Cadmium compounds Metam sodium Paraquat Diquat Acrolein Chloropicrin Sulfur dioxide Naphthalene Formaldehyde Ethylene oxide Methyl bromide Endothall Toluene Xylene	Thiophthalimides Thiram Thiocarbamates Pentachlorophenol Chlorophenoxy compounds Chlorothalonil Picloram Creosote Aliphatic acids
Tearing	Organophosphates Carbamate insecticides Chloropicrin Acrolein	Pentachlorophenol Pyrethrins
Yellow schlerae	Nitrophenols	Agents that cause jaundice (see above under Skin)
Keratitis	Paraquat	
Ptosis	Thallium	
Diplopia	Organophosphates Carbamate insecticides Nicotine	
Photophobia		Organotin compounds
Constricted visual fields	Organic mercury	
Optic atrophy		Thallium
Miosis	Organophosphates Carbamate insecticides	Nicotine (early)
Dilated pupils	Cyanide Fluoride	
Unreactive pupils	Cyanide	

Nervous System

MANIFESTATION	CHARACTERISTIC OF THESE POISONINGS	OCCURS WITH THESE AGENTS
Paresthesia (chiefly facial, transitory)	Organophosphates Cyanopyrethroids Phosphides Organochlorines Thiabendazole	Nicotine (late)
Paresthesia of extremities	Inorganic arsenicals Organic mercury Sodium fluoroacetate Carbon disulfide Thallium	Pyrethroids (transitory)
Headache	Organophosphates Carbamate insecticides Nicotine Inorganic arsenicals Organic mercury Cadmium compounds Organotin compounds Copper compounds Thallium Fluoride Borates Naphthalene Phosphine Halocarbon fumigants Creosote Diquat Cholecalciferol Cyanamide	Organochlorines Nitrophenols Thiram Pentachlorophenol Paraquat Diethyltoluamide
Behavioral – mood Disturbances (confusion, excitement, mania, disorientation, emotional lability)	Organic mercury Inorganic arsenicals Organotin compounds Thallium Nicotine Sodium fluoroacetate Diquat Cyanide Nitrophenols Aminopyridine Carbon disulfide Methyl bromide	Organophosphates Carbamate insecticides Pentachlorophenol Sodium fluoride Diethyltoluamide Organochlorines
Depression, stupor, coma, respiratory failure, often without convulsions	Organophosphates Carbamate insecticides Sodium fluoride Borate Diquat	Inorganic arsenicals Metaldehyde Sulfuryl fluoride Halocarbon fumigants Phosphorus Phosphine Paraquat Chlorophenoxy compounds Diethyltoluamide Alkyl phthalates

Nervous System (continued)

MANIFESTATION	CHARACTERISTIC OF THESE POISONINGS	OCCURS WITH THESE AGENTS
Seizures/Convulsions (clonic-tonic) sometimes leading to coma	Organochlorines Strychnine Crimidine Sodium fluoroacetate Nicotine Cyanide Acrylonitrile Metaldehyde Thallium DEET Chlorobenzilate Carbon disulfide Phosphine Povidone-iodine Hexachlorophene Sodium chlorate Creosote Endothall Fluoride	Nitrophenols Pentachlorophenol Inorganic arsenicals Organotin compounds Diquat Borate Sulfuryl fluoride Methyl bromide Chlorophenoxy compounds Organophosphates Carbamate insecticides Aminopyridine
Muscle twitching	Organophosphates Carbamate insecticides Nicotine Sulfuryl fluoride	Organic mercury Chlorophenoxy compounds
Myotonia		Chlorophenoxy compounds
Tetany, carpopedal spasms	Fluoride Phosphides Phosphorus	
Tremor	Organic mercury Thallium Organophosphates Carbamate insecticides Nicotine Metaldehyde Borates	Pentachlorophenol Nitrophenole Thiram
Incoordination (including ataxia)	Halocarbon fumigants Organophosphates Carbamate insecticides Carbon disulfide Nicotine Thallium	Organic mercury Organochlorines
Paralysis Paresis, muscle weakness	Inorganic arsenicals Organophosphates Carbamate insecticides Nicotine	Organic mercury Diethyltoluamide
Hearing loss	Organic mercury	

Nervous System (continued)

MANIFESTATION	CHARACTERISTIC OF THESE POISONINGS	OCCURS WITH THESE AGENTS
Hypotension shock	Phosphorus Phosphides Phosphine Sodium fluoride Sodium chlorate Borate Thallium Copper compounds Endothall Cyanamide	Inorganic arsenicals Nicotine (late) Creosote Alkyl phthalate Cycloheximide Formaldehyde Norbormide
Hypertension	Thallium (early) Nicotine (early)	Organophosphates

Cardiovascular System

MANIFESTATION	CHARACTERISTIC OF THESE POISONINGS	OCCURS WITH THESE AGENTS
Cardiac arrhythmias	Sodium fluoroacetate Halocarbon fumigants Nicotine Sodium fluoride Ethylene oxide Sodium chlorate Thallium-ventricular Povidone-iodine Veratrum alkaloid (sabadilla)	Inorganic arsenicals Phosphorus Phosphides Phosphine Organochlorines Cyanide Acrylonitrile Fluoride
Bradycardia (sometimes to asystole)	Cyanide Organophosphates Carbamate insecticides	Nicotine
Tachycardia	Nitrophenols Pentachlorophenol Cyanamide	Metaldehyde Organophosphates

Respiratory System

MANIFESTATION	CHARACTERISTIC OF THESE POISONINGS	OCCURS WITH THESE AGENTS
Upper respiratory tract irritation, rhinitis, scratchy throat, cough	Naphthalene Paraquat Chloropicrin Acrolein Dichloropropene Ethylene dibromide Sulfur dioxide Sulfuryl fluoride Acrylonitrile Formaldehyde Cadmium dusts ANTU	Dry formulation of copper, tin, zinc compounds Dusts of thiocarbamate and other organic pesticides Chlorophenoxy compounds Aliphatic acides Rotenone
Sneezing	Sabadilla	
Runny nose	Pyrethrins Inorganic arsenicals Organophosphates Carbamate insecticides	Dry formulation of copper, tin, zinc compounds Dusts of thiocarbamate and other organic pesticides Chlorophenoxy compounds Aliphatic acides Rotenone
Pulmonary edema (many chemicals come packaged in a hydrocarbon vehicle, well known to cause pulmonary edema)	Methyl bromide Phosphine Phosphorus Phosphine Ethylene oxide Ethylene dibromide Acrolein Pyrethiods Sulfur dioxide Cationic detergents Creosote Methylisothiocyanate Cadmium	Organophosphates Carbamate insecticides Paraquat Phosphides
Pulmonary consolidation	Paraquat Cadmium dusts Methyl bromide	Diquat
Dyspnea	Organophosphates Carbamate insecticides Nicotine Paraquat ANTU Cadmium dusts Cyanamide Sulfuryl fluoride Pentachlorophenol Methyl bromide Sulfur dioxide Chloropicrin	Nitrophenols Cyanide Creosote Pyrethins

Gastrointestinal Tract and Liver

MANIFESTATION	CHARACTERISTIC OF THESE POISONINGS	OCCURS WITH THESE AGENTS
Nausea, vomiting, commonly followed by diarrhea	Organophosphates Carbamate insecticides Nicotine Arsenicals Fluoride Cadmium compounds Organotin compounds Copper compounds Sodium chlorate Borate Cyanide Chlorophenoxy compounds Phosphorus Phosphides Phosphine Carbon disulfide Chloropicrin Halocarbon fumigants Endothall Metaldehyde Thallium Red quill Diquat Naphthalene Methyl bromide Dibromochloropropane Veratrum alkaloid Thiram	Pentachlorophenol *B.thuringiensis* Cholecalciferol Thiram Ethylene dichloride Propane Ethylene oxide Cresol Many pesticides have some irritant property
Diarrhea (first)	Organophosphates Carbamates Pyrethoids Borates Sulfur Nicotine *B.thuringiensis* Thiram Cadmium	Cationic detergents Cresol Hexachlorophene Chlorophenoxy compounds
Diarrhea (bloody)	Fluoride Paraquat Diquat Thallium Coumarins Indandiones Endothall Arsenicals	Phosphorus Phosphides Cycloheximide

Gastrointestinal Tract and Liver (continued)

MANIFESTATION	CHARACTERISTIC OF THESE POISONINGS	OCCURS WITH THESE AGENTS
Abdominal pain	Organophosphates Carbamate insecticides Paraquat Diquat Nicotine Methaldehyde Fluoride Borate Phosphorous Phosphides Inorganic arsenicals Cadmium compounds Copper compounds Thallium Organotin compounds	Chlorophenoxy compounds Aliphatic acids Sodium chlorate Creosote Endothall Aminopyridine Coumarins Indandiones Fumigants (ingested) Cycloheximide
Stomatitis	Inorganic arsenicals Paraquat Diquat Copper compounds	Thallium
Salivation	Organophosphates Carbamate insecticides Nicotine Aminopyridine Sodium fluoride Cyanide Cadmium compounds	
Ileus	Thallium Diquat	

Liver

MANIFESTATION	CHARACTERISTIC OF THESE POISONINGS	OCCURS WITH THESE AGENTS
Enlargement	Copper compounds Sodium chlorate Phosphine Carbon tetrachloride Cholorform	Inorganic arsenicals Hexachlorobenzene
Jaundice – see section on Skin		

Kidney

MANIFESTATION	CHARACTERISTIC OF THESE POISONINGS	OCCURS WITH THESE AGENTS

Proteinuria
Hematuria
Sometimes leading
  to oliguria
Acute renal failure with
  azotemia
	Inorganic arsenicals
	Copper compounds
	Sodium fluoride
	Naphthalene
	Borate
	Nitrophenols
	Pentacholorphenol
	Sodium chlorate
	Sulfuryl fluoride
	Paraquat
	Diquat
	Arsine
	Ethylene dibromide
		Cadmium compounds
		Phosphorus
		Phosphides
		Phosphine
		Chlorophenoxy compounds
		Creosote
		Organotin compounds

Dysuria, hematuria, pyuria	Chlordimeform	
Polyuria	Cholecalciferol	Fluoride
Hemoglobinuria	Naphthalene Sodium chlorate Arsine	
Wine-red urine (porphyrinuria	Hexachlorobenzene	
Smoky urine	Creosote	
Glycosuria		Organotin compounds
Ketonuria		Borate

Reproductive System

MANIFESTATION	CHARACTERISTIC OF THESE POISONINGS	OCCURS WITH THESE AGENTS
Low sperm count	Dibromochloropropane	Kepone

Blood

MANIFESTATION	CHARACTERISTIC OF THESE POISONINGS	OCCURS WITH THESE AGENTS
Hemolysis	Naphthalene Sodium chlorate Arsine	Copper compounds Cresol
Methemoglobinemia	Sodium chlorate Creosote	Chlordimeform Cyanide Cresol Copper Arsine
Hypoprothrombinemia	Coumarins Indandiones	Phosphorus Phosphides Carbon tetrachloride
Hyperkalemia	Sodium chlorate Naphthalene Arsine	Sodium fluoride
Hypocalcemia	Fluoride	Thallium Phosphorus Phosphides
Hypercalcemia	Cholecalciferol	
Carboxyhemoglobinemia		Organotin compounds
Anemia	Naphthalene Sodium chlorate Arsine Inorganic arsenicals	
Leukopenia, Thrombocytopenia	Inorganic arsenicals	
Elevated LDH GOT, GPT, alkaline phosphatase, ALT, AST enzymes	Carbon tetrachloride Chloroform Phosphine	Inorganic arsenicals Phosphorus Phosphides Phosphine Sodium chlorate Nitrophenols Pentachlorophenol Thallium Organochlorines Chlorophenoxy compounds
Depressed RBC Acetylcholinesterase and plasma pseudocholinesterase	Organosphosphates	Carbamate insecticides

Index of Pesticide Products